# Communication and Interpersonal Skills

# HEALTH AND SOCIAL CARE TITLES AVAILABLE FROM LANTERN PUBLISHING LTD

| ISBN | Title |
|---|---|
| 9781908625144 | A Handbook for Student Nurses |
| 9781908625281 | Caring for People with Learning Disabilities |
| 9781906052041 | Clinical Skills for Student Nurses° |
| 9781906052027 | Effective Management in Long-term Care Organisations |
| 9781906052140 | Essential Study Skills for Health and Social Care |
| 9781906052171 | First Health and Social Care |
| 9781906052102 | Fundamentals of Diagnostic Imaging |
| 9781906052133 | Fundamentals of Nursing Care |
| 9781906052119 | Improving Students' Motivation to Study |
| 9781906052188 | Interpersonal Skills for the People Professions |
| 9781908625021 | Leadership in Health and Social Care |
| 9781906052096 | Neonatal Care |
| 9781906052164 | Palliative Care |
| 9781906052201 | Professional Practice in Public Health |
| 9781906052089 | Safe & Clean Care |
| 9781906052157 | The Care and Wellbeing of Older People |
| 9781906052225 | The Care Process |
| 9781906052218 | Understanding and Helping People in Crisis |
| 9781906052010 | Understanding Research and Evidence-Based Practice |
| 9781908625007 | Understanding Wellbeing |
| 9781906052058 | Values for Care Practice |
| 9781908625229 | Wellbeing: Policy and Practice |

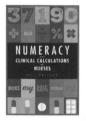 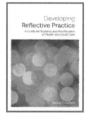 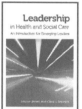 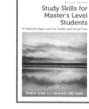 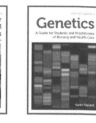

9781908625243    9781908625014    9781908625021    9781908625175    9781908625151

# Communication and Interpersonal Skills

Erica Pavord
and Elaine Donnelly

Lantern

kH

**ISBN 978 1 908625 32 8**

First edition published in 2008 by Reflect Press Ltd (ISBN 9781906052065)

Second edition published in 2015 by Lantern Publishing Limited

Lantern Publishing Limited, The Old Hayloft, Vantage Business Park, Bloxham Rd, Banbury, OX16 9UX, UK

**www.lanternpublishing.com**

**www.cla.co.uk**

**British Library Cataloguing in Publication Data**

A catalogue record for this book is available from the British Library

The authors and publisher have made every attempt to ensure the content of this book is up to date and accurate. However, healthcare knowledge and information is changing all the time so the reader is advised to double-check any information in this text on drug usage, treatment procedures, the use of equipment, etc. to confirm that it complies with the latest safety recommendations, standards of practice and legislation, as well as local Trust policies and procedures. Students are advised to check with their tutor and/or mentor before carrying out any of the procedures in this textbook.

Typeset by Medlar Publishing Solutions Pvt Ltd, India

Cover design by Andrew Magee Design Ltd

Printed in the UK

Distributed by NBN International, 10 Thornbury Rd, Plymouth, PL6 7PP, UK

3/2/16

# CONTENTS

Introduction                                                          vii

About the authors                                                     xi

1  Introducing key concepts in communication                          1

2  Understanding ourselves and our impact on others                  19

3  Interpersonal communication                                       37

4  Introducing Transactional Analysis                                61

5  Listening to people                                               77

6  Communication and interpersonal skills in practice                99

7  Case study                                                       117

   Index                                                            125

# INTRODUCTION

## HELLO AND WELCOME TO THE SECOND EDITION OF THIS BOOK

This is the second edition of this book and it has been revised and updated since the first edition was published in 2008. Two chapters have been replaced by new ones, one has changed significantly and the other chapters have been edited to accommodate the changes. We hope that you continue to find it a useful companion to your studies.

The book itself does not profess to be the definitive text – it is far too small to be that – but what it does do is present and explore some of the key issues and theories that surround effective communication. It explores what happens when communication goes wrong and outlines some possible solutions that you can put in place to limit the consequences of poor communication and to develop more successful communication systems. Good communication is the key to effective care and we hope that you enjoy developing and practising the skills presented here.

We envisaged that our readers would all be students new to the areas of study that surround health and social care and that they would be involved in working across a broad range of health and social care facilities and with a broad mix of people. The authors, who have an interest in the teaching of communication and interpersonal skills, have developed an introductory text that explores communication as a 'skilled behaviour' for students working with people and is based on real teaching and learning activities that have been tried and tested in the classroom.

## WHO IS THIS BOOK FOR?

This book is primarily written to support students undertaking study in any field of health and social care. You may be studying single modules aimed at developing your communication and interpersonal skills or you may be studying a full course for health and social care practitioners such as a Degree course in Nursing and Midwifery, a Foundation Degree in Health and Social Care, a course in Social Work, a course designed for practitioners working in the Hospital and Emergency Care Services, and so on. Regardless of which programme of study you are undertaking, this book is written to provide you with a valuable introduction to the fascinating field of Interpersonal and Communication Skills and it will help you to meet the learning outcomes of your course.

## WHAT DOES THE BOOK COVER?

Like many books in any subject it begins by offering definitions, and then explores the meaning of what it is to be a skilled communicator. We explore simple everyday issues such as courtesy and protocols and what can happen when we forget to apply these in practice. It will introduce you to two theories of communication and give you examples of how the theories relate to practice.

*Chapter 1* provides an overview of what is to come. Like most academic texts the book begins with an examination of definitions and then introduces you to some of the incredibly complex phenomena that surround communication and interpersonal skills.

*Chapter 2* deals with intrapersonal communication and self-awareness; in order for us to understand how to communicate more effectively with others, we need to know ourselves and know why we might respond in different ways to different people. This chapter will encourage you to reflect on who you are, what values and beliefs you have and how these might impact on your communication with others. You will be encouraged to become reflective practitioners, having the ability to reflect on your practice in order to improve your interpersonal skills.

*Chapter 3* takes you on to focus on some of the key issues involved in communication with others. It focuses on interpersonal communication. It looks at the kind of communication that happens both verbally and non-verbally and it explores how different environments can communicate to the people in them and how environments can impact on the way that practitioners and service users communicate. The chapter then discusses the issues relating to intercultural communication and how age, gender, ethnicity and religion affect how we interact with others.

*Chapter 4* focuses on a psychological perspective of intrapersonal communication and interpersonal skills. It introduces the work of Eric Berne and uses Transactional Analysis as a working theory to help you understand your own intrapersonal communication processes and the communications that you have with others.

*Chapter 5* introduces the skills needed to ensure that we are listening in an active and empathic way to the people that we are caring for. Effective communication is largely dependent on our ability to really listen to people and show them that they have been heard and understood. It will describe the Rogerian, person-centred qualities of empathy, acceptance and genuineness and show how to use active listening skills to communicate these qualities to those in our care.

*Chapter 6* encourages you to think about how we communicate with our colleagues and other professionals and touches on the other modes of communication that you will have to use like record-keeping, email, text, mobile phone and social media.

*Chapter 7* gives you a detailed case study which will help you to reflect on the experience of care. It shows the problems involved with dealing with difficult people and gives useful advice on how to manage these situations.

## STUDYING WITH THIS BOOK

The writing team recognises that personal review, self-awareness and reflection can act as a powerful tool in the process of learning and you will be encouraged to reflect on a series of situations and then project the principles learned through these reflections onto your own working experience.

You will then be invited to explore different aspects of interpersonal communication and think about how you can develop your interpersonal skills to ensure that you are working ethically and communicating effectively. Where possible we have provided details of relevant online resources, taking care to include those aspects that relate to the nature of the work that you do and recommending only *bona fide* websites for downloads.

As you read through each chapter you will be invited to supplement your reading with a variety of activities. There are a number of different types of activity in this book.

**READING ACTIVITIES**

Reading activities may involve you looking for and accessing a specific document or text relevant to your place of work or subject area of study. If the reading activity requires you to access detail from the internet we will provide an online web address. We may also encourage you to follow links provided via that address but, again, this is subject to your area of interest. We recognise that some of your supplementary study will be very specific to the area in which you work and the nature of the people you will be working with. To meet your needs we have, where possible, provided alternative online web addresses for you to select from. Sometimes these web addresses change but it is usually possible to find a document by putting its title into a search engine.

Reflecting on what you already know or have had experience of can be a powerful tool in helping you identify what you did and why you did something in a given situation. Reflection on your actions and reflection during your actions can help you to integrate new learning and enable you to become more effective in what you do. Reflective activities may also involve you being asked to imagine something relevant to the topic and to work your way through the same as if it were a real event. *Chapter 2* will introduce you to two useful reflective models that will support your learning.

For writing activities it would be helpful to have a pen and paper to hand to jot down notes or make lists to refer back to at a later point. Writing activities may also be involved in reading and reflecting activities. Some of the activities detailed above may invite you to share your thoughts and ideas with other people and have discussions about key elements of the subject being studied.

Whatever activity is suggested it is completely up to you as to how you study that particular concept. The text and information on these pages will come alive only when you interact with them. So, welcome to this book and enjoy your study of Communication and Interpersonal Skills.

*Erica Pavord and Elaine Donnelly*

# ABOUT THE AUTHORS

**Elaine Donnelly**, before her retirement in 2011, was a Senior Lecturer in Health, Social Care and Psychology at the University of Worcester. Much of her teaching was within the field of nursing and she had previously worked as a mental health nurse in a variety of mental health facilities including elderly care, acute psychiatry and the community. As a registered mental health nurse she was always interested in what makes people behave as they do. Her first degree was in Psychology and she then undertook a Master of Science degree in Health and Social Care. Her research and teaching interests include communication and interpersonal skills, supporting student learning, psychology, psychological development, caring for dying people and their families and supporting the bereaved. As a teacher she had a facilitative style in the classroom, encouraging students to learn through their experience, from each other and through the process of reflection. This was her first venture in writing for publication and she wrote the text in a similar way to her teaching style.

**Erica Pavord** has written the new chapters in this second edition and, with Elaine's blessing has edited and changed the other chapters. Erica works part time as a counsellor for children, young people and their families. Before becoming a counsellor she spent 15 years as a secondary school teacher and has managed to keep the teaching part of her career going by lecturing at Worcester University. In 2010 she took on the teaching of Therapeutic Communication and Interpersonal Skills to Foundation Degree students in Health and Social Care, Mental Health and Child and Adolescent Mental Health. More recently the module was delivered to BSc students in Occupational Therapy and Physiotherapy. The changes in this second edition reflect the development of the module which Erica has continued to teach alongside her colleagues in Worcester. Their contribution to some of the material in this edition has been invaluable.

# 01

# INTRODUCING KEY CONCEPTS
# IN COMMUNICATION

**KEY THEMES:**

- The importance of communication
- Moving towards a definition of communication
- Academic definitions
- Communications theory
- Models of communication.

Being able to communicate effectively is essential for any practitioner working with people. Good communication is central to providing good care and service. This book aims to launch you on an exploration of what it is to communicate effectively with others and the impact that good and bad communication has on the process of care.

## THE IMPORTANCE OF GOOD COMMUNICATION

"Communication underpins all else we do. Effective communication is a two way process which develops and cements relationships, keeps people informed and reduces the likelihood of errors and mistakes."

(NHS Employers, 2014, p. 2)

"Good communication is central to working with children, young people, families and carers. It helps build trust, and encourages them to seek advice and use services. It is key to establishing and maintaining relationships, and is an active process that involves listening, questioning, understanding and responding."

(Children's Workforce Development Council, 2010, p. 6)

Communication is central to everything we do in health and social care. Effective communication is the key to delivering high-quality help and care, regardless of your field or the setting you work in. If any of our communication skills are poor or deficient or if we are negligent in communicating something that is important, the people we aim to care for will be disadvantaged and may suffer in consequence. Constantly reviewing, maintaining and improving your communication skills is a very important part of your work not just as a student but also as a professional. Good communication is not always easy so it is important for you to know a little about the basics of good communication to aid your reflections and study of how to improve your communication/interpersonal skills.

Effective communication is recognised as a core competence for all people who work in public service. The failings in care at the Mid Staffordshire NHS Foundation Trust were documented in the Francis Report (Mid Staffordshire NHS Foundation Trust, 2013) which highlighted the need for a patient-centred and compassionate service for patients. It stated that nursing staff should be recruited in line with core values and behaviours termed the '6 Cs'. These values and behaviours are not new but are put together to reflect the values and beliefs that underpin care wherever it takes place.

## THE 6 Cs

The 6 Cs are:

**Care** – all nurses, midwives and care staff commit to look after patients with **care**.

**Compassion** – all pledge to deliver care with **compassion**, empathy, kindness, trust, respect and dignity.

**Competence** – there is an assurance that this care will be delivered by **competent** nurses, midwives and care staff who have the relevant knowledge, skills and education and who receive ongoing training and support.

**Communication** – all promise that there will be improved **communication** with patients as partners in their care, recognising that communication at a time of vulnerability will always be remembered.

**Courage** – all promise that care will be delivered with the **courage** to speak up when things are wrong, to spread good practice, to challenge, to say stop and to place the interests of others before one's own.

**Commitment** – all staff will make a **commitment** to work as a team and make this care happen for every patient, all day every day. (NHS England, 2013)

Communication is at the foundation of each of the 6 Cs, enabling health and social care workers to demonstrate care and compassion, listening to those we care for and to our colleagues and speaking up when we feel we need to. It is at the heart of effective teamwork, ensuring that everyone works together to provide the best care possible.

**READING ACTIVITY** 1.1

Find and read one of the following documents that is relevant to your field of work or study. As you read, make notes about how you think the document demonstrates how important good communication is.

The document *Compassion in Practice: Nursing Midwifery and Care Staff. Our Vision and Strategy* gives detailed information about the 6 Cs. This can be found at: www.england.nhs.uk/wp-content/uploads/2012/12/compassion-in-practice.pdf

If you are studying to work in any social setting that involves children and young people, find and read the policy document *The Common Core of skills and knowledge*. This is available online at: http://webarchive.nationalarchives.gov.uk/20120119192332/http:/cwdcouncil.org.uk/common-core

If you are studying to work in any NHS setting you should download and read *The NHS Knowledge and Skills Framework*, which helps to guide development and identify the knowledge and skills that you will need in your job. A simplified version can be found at: www.nhsemployers.org/SimplifiedKSF

If you are studying to work within adult social care you should download and read Skills for Care's *Common Induction Standards*, which are the standards people working in adult social care need to meet before they can safely work unsupervised. These can be found at: www.skillsforcare.com/Standards/Common-Induction-Standards/Common-Induction-Standards.aspx

Now that you have read the document most relevant to your field of study, have a look at the other documents and compare the detail. You will find lots of other interesting links that may be useful later on within your studies. You will have found that all the documents have effective communication as a 'core condition' of working with people.

## TOWARDS A DEFINITION OF COMMUNICATION

There are numerous definitions of communication in the *Oxford English Dictionary*. So where should we begin? Before pinning it down to specific definitions, let's begin by looking at what we understand, within the broader context, communication to be.

**WRITING ACTIVITY** 1.1

1. Jot down your own understanding of what the term 'communication' means.
2. Based on what you have jotted down, try to shape those ideas into a working definition.

Creating a succinct definition that takes into account everything you have noted is difficult and you could try to compare your notes with what your fellow students have written. Are there any comparisons to be made or are your definitions completely different?

## My definition of communication

My initial list of what the term 'communication' means was very long. It is what this whole book is all about but, when I came to determine my own definition, my thoughts immediately focused on the notion that communication is about any interaction we have with others. This seemed nice and simple on the surface but as I started to tease the definition out I found several issues that needed to be worked through. The use of the word 'any' creates difficulty for me in exploring what I want to focus on and the use of the word 'others' over-complicates things too.

'Others' could be animals or other living things. I have been known to share my innermost thoughts with my cat (thank goodness he cannot repeat these to other people) and I have been seen talking to plants and vegetables in the garden. At the time of writing I am talking to my computer, not that it ever responds, and perhaps that is the key. I decided to keep my definition simple and, in the context of this book, I define it to be any interaction that takes place between people.

Even though I have tried to keep it simple my definition is still very complicated. Our interactions don't just take place face to face, they take place on many different levels and we use a variety of different methods and many modes of delivery in getting our message across. So, the rider to my definition is that 'communication' is a very difficult term to pin down to one simple statement. When studying definitions of communication it is important to remember that definitions reflect the interest and background of the person making the definition, and may also reflect their perceptions and experiences, so, therefore, their definition is not necessarily true in every context.

## How do we communicate?

So my next thoughts turn to the question of how we communicate. I have no doubt that you have considered this in your response to the writing activity. Communication can be anything from a personal text message from a friend, to a public advertisement on the side of a bus. It might be as simple as a smile or something as technically complicated as a piece of software for a computer. Thinking about methods and modes and channels of communication is an important aspect of understanding what we mean by communication and this is explored further later in this chapter.

When we come to study communication it quickly becomes clear just how complex a phenomenon it is, even though we all engage in it from the minute that we are conceived. On a personal level we communicate with the world around us by the things that we say, the way that we say them, and the things that we do and the way that do them. It can be the clothes we wear, how we style our hair, the way we walk, the way we talk, the way we behave, and how we demonstrate our attitude to life. Communication is all of these things and much more.

## Communication, values and wellbeing

Communication affects the way we feel about ourselves as well as the way we feel about others. According to Littlejohn and Foss (2005), how we communicate is associated with "personal values", with our "culture" and how we "value others" as well as ourselves. We live in a multicultural society and we cannot just consider how we communicate (meaning ourselves within our own cultural group) – we must consider others and how they communicate too. *The NHS Knowledge and Skills Framework* that you read earlier makes it quite clear that Communication (Core Dimension 1) is very closely linked with Equality and Diversity (Core Dimension 6). *The Common Core of skills and knowledge* for the Children's Workforce also makes it clear that communication is closely linked with ethical practice and respect for ourselves and others.

Psychologists study communication and have argued that at every age and stage of our lives communication is fundamental to our very being. We all have different levels at which we feel comfortable communicating but we all need to do so to keep us well and functioning (West and Turner, 2007). According to Bowlby (1969) and Crowley and Hunter (2005), in situations where human beings are isolated and consequently forced into non-communication, their mental and physical health deteriorate. In tiny babies non-communication can lead to very severe consequences and be life threatening (Bowlby, 1969).

I am confident that as a result of the writing activity above you are now aware of just how big a subject communication is and, as our main focus is interpersonal skills and communicating with others, perhaps you are now able to summarise this discussion and, as a result, would like to review your own definition before moving on to look at the definitions of others.

## Definitions in academic study

In academic study it is always more useful to explore subject-specific definitions or, at least, definitions written by scholars within a particular discipline. Take the following definition, for example. Wood (2004) defines communication as "a process in which individuals interact with and through symbols to create and interpret meaning". On the surface this could be viewed simply as a collection of words but there are many levels on which you can explore this definition. Let us look at those words and how Wood explains her perceptions and understanding of what communication is. The definition uses the word 'process', which is commonly understood to be a series of actions or activities that produce something. The word 'individuals' suggests not just communicating with oneself but also with others. So communication, according to this definition, is about taking part or sharing actions with another person or with a group of people.

## Symbols

Wood (2004) suggests that we use 'symbols' in our communication with ourselves and with others and that we 'create' and 'interpret meaning' through those symbols. This throws another interesting perspective into the definition. 'Symbols' are things that represent something else. They can be in the form of a material object, such as your country's national flag, or they could be in the form of a symbolic action such as a gesture.

Alongside this idea we need to put the notion that we then 'create' and 'interpret meanings' from such symbolism, either through a shared activity or via our own internal understanding. That seems relatively simple but the creation and interpretation of symbols can present us with all sorts of difficulty because symbols can be interpreted differently by different people and their use in communication can be a little precarious.

**REFLECTION** 1.1

1. Have in front of you a small piece of paper, approximately 2 inches by 3 inches (5 cm by 7.5 cm), and colour it in red. Paint, felt tip or crayon will do nicely. Look at that piece of red paper. Does it mean anything to you?

2. Now imagine yourself holding that small piece of red paper above your head in a busy supermarket. Would the action of holding up your art work mean anything to the people around you? How do you think people would react to you? How do you think you would feel?

It is more than likely that people would perceive you as a little 'odd' and, consequently, having had a little peek at you (we are all curious beings after all) the people around you would ignore you and get on with their shopping and perhaps you would be left feeling a little foolish.

Now imagine that you are a referee on a football pitch. That little piece of red paper, all of a sudden, takes on new meaning. It has a symbolic function. It is seen as a Red Card. The Red Card symbolises that one of the players is judged by the referee to be guilty of a serious misdemeanour and is to be sent off the pitch. If you were the referee it is likely that you wouldn't feel foolish in this situation at all; rather you would feel noticed, validated, powerful and in charge. Although, perhaps, my perceptions of what it is to be a referee are a little at odds with reality. But whose reality? This is an important issue. It seems that we all share common realities and understand symbols that are meaningful to us but each of us also has our own interpretations of the world and these interpretations are influenced by some of the factors that Littlejohn and Foss (2005) outline in relation to values, social groups and culture.

I am going to follow this through a little more as it raises important issues for us to understand. If we were observers of the football match, regardless of how big the stadium was or how many people were there, we would easily spot a small piece of red card in the hand of the man dressed in black, and we instantly recognise the meaning of the action and the symbolism of the card. Knowing the Red Card's function we will respond, but our response isn't always absolutely predictable, even if we all interpreted the symbolic action the same way. Our response to observing the Red Card will be in accordance with whether or not we support the referee's decision to give a Red Card. Our interpretation of the referee's action is likely to reflect where our support lies; is it someone on our own team who is being sent off or someone on the opposite side? Our response could be predicted by the colour of the team colours or scarf that we wear and/or by the end of the stadium at which we stand or sit while the game is being played. However, our responses to symbols are not always this clear cut.

So, something as simple as a Red Card triggers all sorts of communications and interactions among people. We all see the same symbol and we all understand the meaning, but we interpret the referee's behaviour differently. Some of us may cheer ecstatically while others boo and jeer as loudly as possible, and then there are those who would go on to discuss the ins and outs of the decision for ever (can you detect from my communication that I dislike post mortems of football matches? How did you detect that?).

**REFLECTION**  1.2

1. Can you think of other examples of symbols and symbolic actions in everyday life and how we attribute meaning to them?
2. How does that attribution of meaning influence our behaviour?
3. What are the possible consequences of symbols and symbolic actions being misinterpreted by others?

I'm sure that you were able to think of many circumstances where symbols influence your behaviour. Road traffic signs are a good example of how a symbol can influence our behaviour. The speed camera sign always makes me check my speed and traffic signage uses simple symbols to convey a whole host of messages targeted at influencing our driving behaviour. Symbols can create unity and symbols can create tension. Symbolic acts have started wars, sparked revolution and changed lives, and whether those changes were good or bad is down to your interpretation of them.

The definition offered by Wood (2004) raises some essential issues in studying communication that I was not able to raise in my definition earlier. It is important that we stop and make the time to explore definitions and try to see the world as others perceive it to be. It will enrich our understanding and enable us to make more positive decisions about how we communicate. Communication is about who we are. It isn't a single one-off thing. It is a very complicated process and to assist you in understanding some of the complexities involved in communicating with yourself and with others, it has been broken down into different areas of study in *Chapters 2* and *3*.

## MODES OF COMMUNICATION

Messages are communicated in many different ways. New methods of transmission and new channels of communication are developing at an incredibly rapid pace as we progress into the digital age. Over the last 50 years the developments in technology have had a massive impact on how we communicate with each other. We can connect online with someone on the other side of the world in an instant and with someone in space at the flick of a switch. Since the publication of the first edition of this book, smartphones have further revolutionised the way that we connect with others. Information technology has changed the world we live in more than any other technical phenomenon. When studying in any field of health and social care you will find that ICT plays a vital role in how we deliver, record and monitor care. As practitioners in whatever field you work in, you have a responsibility to develop and update your skills accordingly.

**WRITING ACTIVITY** 1.2

> Think of all the different ways your grandparents and your great-grandparents may have communicated with each other and the rest of the world as young people, and draw up a list of these.

If you have the opportunity, speak with a person aged 80 years plus and see if they can confirm the ways you have identified. They may be able to add to your list with some very interesting examples of means of communication. No doubt some of their methods were quite innovative, particularly if they involved speaking with boyfriends and girlfriends without their parents being aware and, of course, communicating during the war years.

Perhaps your list will have included some of the following:
- face-to-face, person-to-person conversation;
- whistling, singing and calling out loud;
- telephone, via the operator of course;
- writing, including letters, postcards, poetry and song;
- handwritten records and ledgers and typed correspondence;
- telegraphy, telegrams and couriers;
- sign language and ticktack, and secret gestures;
- secret codes and messaging banners, flags and semaphore;
- flickering lights, and opening and shutting curtains;
- pigeon post and go-betweens, flares and other pyrotechnics;
- radio, television and cinema.

These are only the examples we could come up with but no doubt there are many more.

**WRITING ACTIVITY** · 1.3

Cover the next section of text and extend your list to include all modes and methods of communication that you have seen or taken part in, either in your personal life or in your experience of work. It is likely to be quite long. Then compare what you have written with the list we have generated below.

- Computers, laptops, tablets;
- Text messaging, email;
- Social media like Facebook, Twitter and Tumblr;
- Telephone (land line), mobile phone and smartphones;
- Blogs and podcasts;
- YouTube;
- Snapchat, Instagram, Kik and Gifboom;
- Satellite communications such as GPS and SatNav;
- Electronic records and online forms;
- Care documentation and care plans;
- Voicemail, pagers, bleeps and alarms;
- Radio waves, X-rays and scans.

This is by no means a comprehensive list and we are sure you can think of others, especially if you are information technology natives. Channels of communication are developing all the time and this requires us to be engaged in learning and developing our skills in communication throughout our lives.

## CHOOSING YOUR APPROACH WHEN COMMUNICATING WITH OTHERS

When communicating directly with people, you first need to choose the mode or the approach that you are going to use and, to be effective in getting your message across, you need to consider some key issues.

**REFLECTION** · 1.3

Imagine yourself in the workplace and being involved in communicating with a person or several people about future plans. What methods or channels of communication might you consider before engaging in that communication? Share your considerations with a colleague.

Your reflection and discussions may have involved you considering some of the following:
- Will the communication be face-to-face, written or using technology?
- Will you use letters, pictures or leaflets in the communication to help clarify what it is you are communicating?

- How much control do you have over the environment and how much control do you have over the timing of the communication?
- How many people are you communicating with and what level of understanding do they have?
- Are there any language or disability issues to consider?
- Do you want people to respond to you and, if so, how do you want them to respond to you?
- Do you want people to have the opportunity to ask questions and how much information do you need to get back from them?
- How detailed should the communication be and how important is this communication at this point?

When communicating with people in the workplace it is important that we think carefully about the channel of communication we use, so that we can make sure we pick the most effective method for them. People are individuals and what is satisfactory for one may be completely inappropriate for another. If you are working with families you may have to use several channels of communication, and to target individual members. A leaflet and a quick explanation may suffice in some circumstances but, in others, we need to employ a wide range of interpersonal and communication skills to ensure that what we do is effective for everyone concerned.

## STUDYING COMMUNICATIONS THEORY

Studying communications theory can help us to understand how communication works and to determine the most effective communication channel to use. Knowing how communication works, we can then understand how, why and where communication goes wrong. When communication goes wrong in health and social care settings the consequences can be far-reaching. People and families can be misjudged, errors in decision-making can be made and care may be seriously compromised, leaving you and the people you care for at risk.

If we can identify how communication takes place and understand its process, we can develop strategies to ensure that communication is effective and meets the needs of all concerned. To help you understand communication we are first going to look at the key frameworks within which the theories and models of communication are set.

### Frameworks of communication

There are four main frameworks for theories of communication. These are:
- **Mechanistic** – this framework was originally used by people working on radio and telephone communications and incorporates a transmission model of communication.

- **Psychological** – this framework concentrates far more on how we feel during a communication and our emotional responses.
- **Social Constructionist** – this framework is concerned with how we all construct different realities from the same experiences. The Symbolic Interaction Theory that we will be looking at is included in this framework.
- **Systemic** – this framework concentrates on the way that communication is part of a whole system and how, within that system, each part of the communication is repeatedly re-examined and reworked.

We are going to look at two models of communication within these frameworks. The first is a Transmission Model. This type of model is included in the Mechanistic Framework and is said to be linear in its process. It is a simple straightforward model that is easy to understand and can be very useful in helping analyse communication processes between people and organisations.

The second model we will look at is a Transactional Model that combines principles from the Psychological, Social Constructionist and Systemic frameworks. The Transactional Model is more complicated than the Mechanistic one and further explores the experience of shared meanings in our communications with others that we discussed earlier. We will then follow an example of a Transactional Model in practice by exploring the psychotherapeutic theory of Transactional Analysis in *Chapter 4*.

## The Shannon and Weaver Transmission Model

One of the earliest, most basic and well-known communication models is that of Shannon and Weaver (1949). Their model is sometimes referred to as the 'Mother of Communication Models' and it provides a good starting point for anyone studying communication theory.

As you can see in *Figure 1.1*, the arrows that show transmission from the Information Source to the Destination point in only one direction, reflecting the belief that messages flow in only one direction at any given time. It is therefore a linear process.

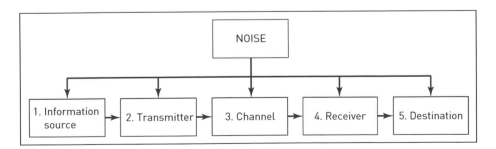

**Figure 1.1** *The Shannon and Weaver Transmission Model.*

The Shannon and Weaver model consists of five parts and what they term 'noise'. In a face-to-face communication
1.  the information would be the idea that you had in your head;
2.  the transmitter would be you sending the message;
3.  the channel would be your voice as you speak the idea;
4.  the receiver would be the ear of the person to whom you are talking;
5.  the destination would be the intended person's head.

Noise, as you can see, can occur at any point within that communication process, and can prevent the original thought or idea reaching its destination intact and as intended. Noise can be anything. Noise might be
*   physical, i.e. what we commonly call noise, a loud sound (physical noise);
*   psychological, i.e. an emotion such as anxiety or a strongly-held point of view or a cultural barrier (psychological noise);
*   semantic, i.e. a language or representation problem (semantic noise);
*   physiological, i.e. deafness, blindness or pain (physiological noise).

Noise can interrupt the communication at any stage.

**REFLECTION** 1.4

1.  Imagine yourself in a busy work area. What sorts of noise do you think might stop your message getting through to another person?
    *   Are people or machines making a 'noise'?
    *   Is the other person in an emotional state, are they flustered, worried, angry or even frightened?
    *   Is their perception of the situation different from yours?
    *   Do they understand the language you are using?
    *   Do they have a particular communication problem?
2.  Make a list of some of the common things that you think would cause 'noise' and interfere with communications in your place of work, and discuss your experiences with a colleague. It might help if you list the noises under the headings offered. You'll be surprised at what constitutes 'noise', particularly when you explore the psychological aspect.

If your message is not getting across, this simple model gives you the opportunity to explore some of the reasons why. Once the 'noise' is identified you can then try to eliminate or at least modify the 'noise' or message in some way. The possibilities are all subject to the nature of the 'noise' and may require you to do some strategic thinking and extra planning to ensure your message gets across. Can you think of any recent examples of 'noise' interfering with a message you wanted to convey? In *Chapters 2* and *6* we will look at noise again by thinking about blocks and barriers to communication and we'll be exploring ways of overcoming these barriers in order to ensure effective communication.

As teachers we experience 'noise' in the learning situation all the time, particularly in the large groups that we sometimes have to teach. We often hear colleagues say, 'I told the students yesterday, why don't they listen?' Our response is always the same. Telling someone something doesn't mean they have heard what you say and, using Shannon and Weaver's model, our approach is to identify the 'noise' that stopped the message getting across and to try other ways to make sure the message is delivered, heard and understood. Other methods to overcome noise in this example will often involve using alternative modes and channels of communication including announcements, notices, ICT, other people, good old repeating oneself, using humour to capture attention, jumping up and down or sometimes even whispering. These are all strategies that we use in the classroom. The strategies you use should be appropriate to the situation and to the person or people you are communicating with. Never believe that people have heard exactly what you meant to say without first checking their understanding and making sure the message reached its destination intact and as you intended it. Using such a simple strategy will help avoid all sorts of complications later on.

## Julia Wood's Transactional Model

The other model of communication to be discussed here is a Transactional Model developed by Julia Wood (2004). Earlier in this chapter we explored her definition of communication. You will recall that communication is:

> "...a systemic process in which individuals interact with and through symbols to create and interpret meanings."
>
> (Wood, 2004)

That definition was then broken down into components for analysis, and part of this discussion explored the significance of symbols in our communication, how they impact upon our behaviour and how we create and interpret meanings through that process.

Wood (2004) offers the following diagram (*Figure 1.2*) to illustrate communications taking place between two people.

In this model you can see that communicator **A** transmits a message to communicator **B**, who receives the message, decodes the message, has a reaction to the message and then responds to communicator **A**. Notice that the 'noise' surrounds the process and that 'shared messages' have a direct impact on the communication between the two.

This is a far more complex model of communication than Shannon and Weaver's which, you will recall, was linear in its process. In this model messages are being sent backwards and forwards all the time, not just in one direction but simultaneously. The Transactional Model focuses on how we interpret meaning and how meanings are shared within our communication with other people.

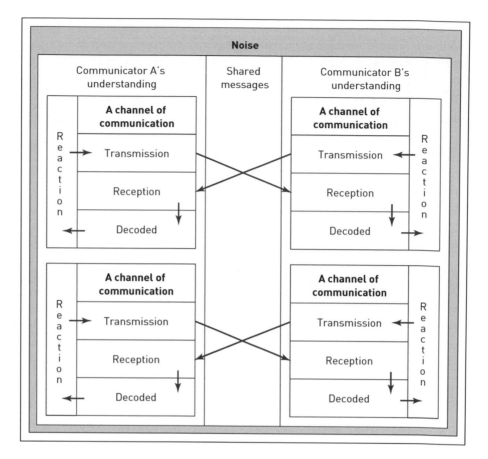

**Figure 1.2** *The Transactional Model.*

When communication goes wrong it is often the result of meaning being misinterpreted. Meaning in communication is said to be negotiated between the people concerned. For example, if you use a word in one context with friends it will be interpreted in a particular way by that social group but, use the same word or communication with your teachers or parents, and the meaning is not shared on the same level. For example, the words 'sick', 'whatever' and 'random' come to mind, as we know older people's interpretations of these words are completely different from those of younger people. There are, no doubt, lots of other examples you can think of. Our language is constantly developing and has to accommodate new ways of living, new technologies and new ways of expressing feelings and thoughts. Social groups use a common language to communicate on a psychological and sociological level that isn't always instantly apparent to people on the outside of that group.

The language we use, our non-verbal behaviours and the symbols we include in our communications all play a powerful role in establishing and sharing meaning. It is important to remember that understanding something is a subjective experience.

We construct meaning in social contexts and share a mutual awareness and often a mutual language that is culturally bound and age-related.

The Transactional Model is a more accurate model of what really happens in face-to-face communication than the Shannon and Weaver model. The Transactional Model takes into consideration all the aspects of communication that we looked at earlier in this chapter. It is also a better basis for any new communication system you might consider creating to help the people you work with. What is it in the Transactional Model that makes it so much better at explaining what real-life communication is like? The answer lies in the channels of communication.

## Channels of communication

In the Transactional Model multiple channels are being used. For example:
- facial expressions;
- body angle;
- posture;
- presentation;
- tone of voice;
- words;
- word images;
- role portrayal.

If you refer back to *Figure 1.2* you will see that not only are multiple channels being used, but the arrows point both ways instead of in just one way. The person sending the message is at the same time receiving a message through the same channels. As each person receives a message they are simultaneously decoding it. They are using all their previous experiences and memories to sift through what they are receiving in order to give meaning to it. At the same time they are creating and sending their own message and there is still all that 'noise' going on around the communications being sent, received and decoded.

There are a number of channels that we use to communicate with others. These channels or methods tend to correspond to particular senses such as sight and hearing and, for each channel that we use, there is a method or way that facilitates its use best. We all communicate in many different forms, and the methods available for us to communicate are always increasing as information and communication technology develops, providing us with the opportunity to use multiple channels of communication to get our messages across. All the channels or methods have different advantages and disadvantages. When choosing a way to communicate, some of the aspects that you need to take into consideration are:
- how much time is available;
- how many people you are communicating with;

- whether you want people to reply to you;
- whether you want people to be able to ask you questions;
- how much information you want to get from them;
- how much information you want to give them;
- how many senses (seeing, hearing, smelling) you need them to use for them to understand the information.

The way we choose to communicate with people depends on the channels of communication open to us. In a normal situation you do not notice yourself deciding on the considerations above when you communicate with someone. However, as someone working in a helping capacity in the health and social care fields, you do need to think more carefully about the best ways to communicate with someone else. You need to take into account their needs and not just yours and balance those needs against the needs of the organisation you work within.

The message here is that once you start to unpick a communication and begin analysing the process you can start to appreciate the depth of meaning that lies behind the words and actions that you engage in. Even if you try not to interact with others you are still communicating with them. By hiding in the sluice or in the back room / office or just by simply staring out of the window you are communicating that you do not wish to interact with them. We communicate with all of our senses, our sight, hearing, smell and touch – in fact, we cannot *not* communicate and in order to ensure that what we are communicating is appropriate, we need to be more consciously aware of the impact we have on others. *Chapter 2* will focus on how we can raise our awareness of ourselves and gain insight into the way that we interact with others.

**CHAPTER SUMMARY**

**Seven key points to take away from Chapter 1:**

- Effective communication is the key to developing and delivering high-quality help and care.
- Policy and legislation indicate that effective communication is a core skill for all people who work in public service.
- It is important that we consider the different methods and modes of communication that we use in different contexts.
- We use 'symbols' in our communication and create and interpret meaning through symbols.
- Modes of communication have changed rapidly over the last 50 years and technology has revolutionised the way that we communicate.

**CHAPTER SUMMARY CONT'D**

- We need to choose the most effective mode or channel of communication when we communicate directly with people, so that our message is conveyed in the most effective way.
- Communications theory can help us to understand how communication works and help us to determine the most effective communication channel to use.

## USEFUL READING

You will already be familiar with the documents listed in *Reading activity 1.1*. If you are interested in finding out more about communications theory, the following books would be useful:

Hargie, O. (1986) *A Handbook of Communication Skills*. London: Routledge.

Littlejohn, S.W. and Foss, K.A. (2005) *Theories of Human Communication*. Belmont, CA: Wadsworth.

Wood, J. (2004) *Communication Theories in Action: An Introduction*. Belmont, CA: Wadsworth/Thomson Learning.

## REFERENCES

Bowlby, J. (1969) *Attachment*. New York: Basic Books.

Children's Workforce Development Council (2010). *The Common Core of skills and knowledge*. Leeds: CWDC.

Crowley, P. and Hunter, J. (2005) Putting the public back into public health. *Journal of Epidemiology and Community Health*, **59**: 265–267.

Littlejohn, S.W. and Foss, K.A. (2005) *Theories of Human Communication*. Belmont, CA: Wadsworth.

Mid Staffordshire NHS Foundation Trust (2013). Available at: www.midstaffs publicinquiry.com/report (accessed 3 February 2015).

NHS (2013) Compassion in Practice – our culture of compassionate care. Available at: www.england.nhs.uk/nursingvision/ (accessed 3 February 2015).

NHS Employers (2014) *Simplified Knowledge and Skills Framework (KSF)*. Available at: www.nhsemployers.org/SimplifiedKSF (accessed 3 February 2015).

Shannon, C. and Weaver, W. (1949) *The Mathematical Theory of Communication*. Urbana, IL: University of Illinois Press.

West, R. and Turner, L.H. (2007) *Introducing Communication Theory: Analysis and application*. New York: McGraw-Hill.

Wood, J. (2004) *Communication Theories in Action: An introduction*. Belmont, CA: Wadsworth/Thomson Learning.

# 02

# UNDERSTANDING OURSELVES AND OUR IMPACT ON OTHERS

**KEY THEMES:**

- Intrapersonal communication
- Self-awareness
- How external and internal factors affect the 'self' that we bring to our practice
- Values and beliefs
- Reflection and reflective practice.

In order to be effective communicators we need to know ourselves and be aware of how our communication impacts on others. In understanding ourselves we are more able to adapt our behaviour and change the effect that we have on others. The much-quoted Socrates said "My friend, care for your psyche, know thyself, for once we know ourselves, we may learn how to care for ourselves"; this chapter encourages you to spend some time thinking about and 'caring' about yourself so that you can become better at thinking about and caring for others.

## INTRAPERSONAL COMMUNICATION

The way we communicate with others is known as interpersonal communication and we will look at that process in *Chapter 3*, but first we will look at this notion of intrapersonal communication. Intrapersonal communication is the communication that we have with ourselves, the self-talk that we engage in on an hour-by-hour basis. As we experience those inner thoughts we also experience feelings which in turn affect how we behave when communicating or making contact with someone else. We have all been in the situation where someone says something to us and it sparks a thought which stops us from listening to the other person because the voice inside our head seems to be talking more loudly.

All of our communication is influenced by how we feel at the time and how we perceive ourselves to be. Intrapersonal communication is a cognitive function in that it relates to our thoughts, but it also plays a significant part in our emotions and how we understand the world to be and our place in it. As humans we self-regulate our behaviour, and the way in which we self-regulate and respond to our innermost feelings and thoughts has an impact on how we present ourselves to the world. Whatever we see, hear, smell or feel as part of that communication is:

- evaluated by our brains based on past knowledge and experience
- reviewed by our senses
- and then evaluated again.

This inner process often continues even after the 'physical communication' has ended. An example of this is when we replay a conversation time and time again in our heads, imagining the different responses that we, and the other people involved, could have made. We often imagine not just what might have been said, but the looks that might have been exchanged, the gestures that we might make, even the emotions we or the other person might feel. The outcome in our head may be completely different from the outcome that was achieved. We have the potential to change the meaning of a comment or interaction completely because we have convinced ourselves of a meaning that makes sense to us and fits with our view of ourselves and others. As professionals we have a responsibility to recognise and understand our *intrapersonal* communication so that we can better reflect on our *interpersonal* communication. We do this by becoming more self-aware and knowing our strengths and limitations.

## SELF-AWARENESS

To be self-aware is to be able to recognise our character traits, our feelings and thoughts and to have insight into how our behaviour is affected by them. Individuals are ultimately responsible for their own input, and developing the skills of self-awareness is the first step to the development of good communication and interpersonal skills. We need to know and understand our own self and to be able to view ourselves from other people's perspectives. We need to be willing to recognise those parts of ourselves that are more or less helpful in our professional roles and be able to change those aspects which get in the way of good communication. There are two important aspects of self-awareness which will be focused on separately; these are awareness of external influences on our sense of self and awareness of internal influences on our sense of self.

## DEVELOPING AWARENESS OF HOW EXTERNAL FACTORS IMPACT ON THE SELF

Often workers in health and social care settings will feel completely exhausted, physically and emotionally and often both. We need to be able to recognise times when we find it hard to communicate effectively because we are feeling physically or emotionally overloaded and unable to give the space and time to someone in our care because we are too full of our own concerns. Physical exhaustion is easier to identify – we usually know when we are tired and hungry, but sometimes it is only when our mood changes and we become less patient and more careless that we realise that our physical needs are being neglected. Unfortunately those around us will have been affected by our short temper or lack of concentration and the quality of our interactions with them will have suffered. It is important for us to be able to pick up on the signs of hunger and tiredness and make sure that we eat regularly and take rest when we can.

If we have behaved in an insensitive or careless way to those we are caring for or working with, we need to have the awareness to recognise it and take steps to repair the relationship. It is not difficult to approach someone and say "I'm sorry I was so short with you this afternoon, I was tired and hungry and I wasn't focusing on your needs." Sometimes a slight rupture in a relationship and the repairing of it can strengthen it; when we know that someone is real and genuine and able to recognise when they have made a mistake, we can feel more trusting of them than if they were perfect all the time.

When the exhaustion is emotional it can be more difficult to recognise. The very nature of the work in health and social care settings is emotionally draining. The people we are caring for need our help, understanding and compassion and sometimes, when we spend all day, every day giving this, we find we might become overwhelmed by the emotional and physical needs of others. We might find that we are unable to listen effectively or compassionately; we get irritated and annoyed easily; we find ourselves crying or shouting at inappropriate times. Health and social care professionals are often surrounded by a supportive and empathic team who are alert to each other's needs, but in busy environments, unless we recognise we are struggling and ask for help directly, our needs sometimes go unnoticed.

In order to minimise the potential for poor communication because of emotional overload, we need to become better at noticing how we are feeling. If we are more aware of what is going on for us emotionally, we are more able to notice when our interactions with others are being affected. Here are some ways in which you can become more aware:
- Take time at the beginning of the day and whenever you have a break to sit and 'check in' with yourself. Breathe deeply and focus on which parts of your body feel tension. Take notice of it and if you know it relates to particular issues which can't be resolved immediately, try to put it somewhere safe (in your mind) to be dealt with later. Very useful techniques for focusing ourselves come from 'mindfulness' and 'mindful practice'. With its roots in Buddhist meditation, mindfulness has entered the mainstream in many diverse settings through the work of

Jon Kabat-Zinn (2004). Mindfulness helps us to deal with emotional overload by becoming more aware of our thoughts and feelings so that instead of becoming overwhelmed by them, we're better able to manage them.

- Talk to someone about your concerns. You should have a colleague, mentor or supervisor with whom you can discuss what you are feeling and the difficulties that you are facing. As we will see in *Chapter 5*, having someone listen to you and focus on you and your concerns can help even if there are no solutions.

- Keep a journal, particularly when you are training, in which you write about your day, the stresses and fun or interesting times. Reflect on how certain situations made you feel and think and reflect on why you might have responded the way you did and how you might respond differently next time. Reflective practice, focused on later in this chapter, is an excellent way to grow in self-awareness.

**REFLECTION** 2.1

Imagine this scenario. A worker in a residential care home is half way through her third night shift in a row. She is particularly exhausted because her 5-year old daughter has been home unwell so she hasn't been able to get much sleep during the day. Her husband has had to cancel his plans so that he can stay at home with their daughter and he is annoyed with her. Her own mother is also unwell and is in hospital having tests. The care home is short staffed so she is having to do more than the usual amount of work. She is called for the fifth time into the room of a new resident who is finding it hard to sleep. It is clear that the resident is physically all right but she is tearful and anxious. The care worker checks on her again and when the resident asks her to stay with her for a few moments, she says "No, I haven't got time, I'm rushed off my feet, there's nothing wrong with you, you aren't the only person I have to look after."

- What are the physical pressures for both the carer and resident?
- What are the emotional pressures for both the carer and resident?
- How have they impacted on the way that the carer communicates?
- What could she have done instead?

## Knowing our limitations

Self-awareness means that we are able to recognise when we are not in a position to do our job as we would like to, or carry out our responsibilities as we are expected to. A typical personality trait of people working in health and social care is a desire to be helpful to others. We have to know when we are not able to help someone in the way that they need and be able to talk to them about alternatives, without feeling that we are letting them down. We also need to be able to tell our colleagues and managers when we feel unable to carry out a particular task or fill a particular role. Muddling through and making do can have damaging consequences for you, the service user and the organisation you are working in. Self-awareness and openness will help you to recognise when you have reached your limits and need to talk to someone else.

# DEVELOPING AWARENESS OF HOW INTERNAL FACTORS IMPACT ON THE SELF

So far we have focused on how an awareness of our physical and emotional needs can help us to think more carefully about how we interact with others. Equally important and influential are more deeply rooted traits which come from our values and beliefs and how they affect our attitudes. Carl Rogers, the father of the person-centred approach to helping relationships, in writing about his own self-awareness said: "The most curious paradox is that when I accept myself just as I am, then I can change." (Rogers, 1961, p. 17.) So, in the spirit of Rogers, this part of the chapter will encourage you to explore who you are and how you came to be you.

## Values and beliefs

A value is something that is worth something or is important to us. Values can have financial or emotional worth and they can be important personally and/or professionally. They can be important to us as individuals or as part of a group. In health and social care we hopefully value ways of being, such as kindness and respect, and values like these guide us in our decision-making, our actions and the way that we interact with others. Values are often formed by certain beliefs that we hold.

Beliefs are assumptions that we make about ourselves, others and the world around us. Many beliefs are held by most cultures in the world: for example most people believe that it is wrong to take another human life or to steal, but all beliefs are dependent on environment and experience. So, there may be some cultures in which individualism and power are valued more than kindness, and these values are held dear by some individuals, families or groups of people within that culture. Whatever our values and beliefs are, they will inevitably affect the way that we communicate with others.

Cuthbert and Quallington (2008) cite Beauchamp and Childress (2001, p. 30) who highlight the values and virtues often associated with healthcare practitioners:

- compassion
- empathy

- sincerity
- discernment
- trustworthiness
- integrity
- conscientiousness
- benevolence and non-malevolence (doing good and not harming)
- truthfulness
- respectfulness.

If these virtues were skills, we could learn and perfect them and we would all be excellent practitioners, but the majority of them are dependent on our own personal beliefs and values; they are often deeply rooted within us and all we can do is become more aware of how they affect us. Sometimes our personal values clash with the professional values we need to uphold. We might all aspire to hold these values but at times they escape us and we feel irritation, anger, impatience or boredom. We might be so exhausted that all we value is sleep and food. There are times when we find it difficult to communicate because we find it hard to like or get on with someone, because their values and beliefs are at such odds to our own. In order to work ethically and to communicate effectively we need to be able to recognise when we find our values and beliefs challenged.

Our values and beliefs are not fixed, they are formed and change throughout our lives and are dependent on where we come from, who we grew up with, who influences us at different times and what happens to us. From the beginning of life we are influenced by family and culture and later we are also influenced by our education, both formal and informal, and by our friends and peer groups.

From the moment we become aware of the messages we are given, we start to form our values. Before we are even verbal we pick up on what is important to our parents. Vygotsky, a theorist who believed that children construct knowledge through social interaction, stated that "through others we become ourselves" (Vygotsky, 1966, p. 43). So, through observation and experience we pick up on our parents' values and they become part of our makeup. For example, a child whose parents value cleanliness has her hands and face wiped many times a day. She is told not to pick things up and not to put them in her mouth, she is encouraged not to make a mess with her toys and not to get her clothes dirty. It is easy to see why cleanliness becomes a deeply rooted value and how that child, on becoming a community nurse in adulthood, might find it very challenging to visit a patient in their home which is messy, chaotic, dusty and dirty. She might find it hard to hide her shock or disapproval and communicate this clearly to the patient, who then feels judged and uncomfortable.

REFLECTION    2.2

How would you, as an interested observer, respond to the following situations?

- The daughter of an elderly man in a care home phones once a month to check how her father is.
- A father tells his 6-year old son that he has to practise the violin for at least three hours a day.
- A child comes to school with a creased and dirty uniform most days.
- A family have a picnic by the side of a river and leave their rubbish there when they leave.

If possible, discuss these situations with other people. How much do your responses differ? What do you notice about your own values and how similar or different they are to the values of others?

Values are not static, they are influenced by experiences throughout our lives and can change significantly as we grow up and form our own identities. Some are deeply entrenched and we defend them fiercely. As we grow up our values are influenced by our culture, which might be shared by those of our family but might be very different. Our cultural identity may be based on heritage, individual circumstances and personal choice and is affected by many different factors: our age, gender, ethnicity, religion, language, country of origin, sexual orientation, socioeconomic status, occupation and more (AAMC, 1999). All these factors influence our values and in turn influence the way that we communicate with others.

It is more often in the workplace that we find our values are challenged, as in our personal lives we are more able to choose to spend time with people who are similar to us. Think about a gay male nurse who has, through experience, fought hard for acceptance and equality in both his family and professional life. He values tolerance and acceptance, the freedom to choose and to express himself as he wishes to. He comes across a patient who uses unpleasant and homophobic language. How might his values be challenged? How far should he tolerate the intolerant and how should he communicate with this patient in an ethical and effective way? Unfortunately there are no definitive answers to these questions but they are always present and must be considered when working in any profession that requires us to form good relationships with others. *Chapters 5* and *6* will offer some ideas about how to deal with situations like these.

Our education, friends, peer groups and our workplace play a significant part in the forming of values which might be different from those of our culture and family. When children reach two or three years of age they often start nursery and so voices outside the family start to be heard. Whereas they have until then been influenced perhaps solely by their family, nursery workers and other children start to become important. Sharing and caring for others will be values promoted strongly in early years settings and if these are similar to those promoted at home, they become assimilated into the child's way of being even when these values are at odds with the child's natural egocentricity. Schools and work settings tend to value hard work, conscientiousness and being a team player and students/workers who adhere to those values tend to do well and receive positive feedback.

As children grow up they are more influenced by their peer group and particularly in adolescence, it becomes more important to form an individual identity away from the family (Erikson, 1995). It is at this point that we start to realise that the values that we hold dear, such as friendship, loyalty and being part of a group, might clash with the ideas of our parents and teachers. The adults might well hold the same values but they see them in different ways and possibly put them lower in the list than the safety of their children, academic success and family. This clash of values is useful to us as we venture into adulthood as we have to learn to negotiate, compromise and reflect on how our personal values relate to those of the people around us.

**REFLECTION** **2.3**

Take some time to think about your own values; these might be values that are deeply rooted in your family and culture or those which you have formed due to your own experience. Choose one which you think is firmly entrenched in you – for better or worse! Now ask yourself the following questions in relation to that value.

- Where did this value come from?
- What impact has holding this value had?
- Is it a value that you want to pass on to your children (if you have any)?
- Is the value shared by all your family/siblings? What happens when family members disagree with certain values?
- Have you questioned this value?
- Think of times when this value has been useful to you and other times when it hasn't.
- How do you think holding this value might impact on you as you develop in your career?
- Have there been any times when your values have clashed with someone else's? What happened and how did you resolve it?

In order to increase your awareness of your values and beliefs and how they might affect your interpersonal skills, try to have discussions with your family and friends about the values that you have and apply the questions above. Our values are closely linked to our beliefs and can have a huge impact on the way that we think. If you have a deeply held belief that the world is a dangerous place, you might value safety and cautiousness and you will reject risk and spontaneity. Your thoughts will be affected by this and you might assume that things are going to go wrong if you take a risk. Inevitably this will affect the way that you interact with others and the way that they view you. As you read on, you will be encouraged to think about how your beliefs and thoughts affect you and others and how reflective practice can greatly enhance your skills.

## NEGATIVE THINKING

Most of us think before we speak, even though we may not be aware of it at the time. The thoughts that precede action are often automatic thoughts that are well rehearsed and often rooted in the values and beliefs we grew up with. For some people automatic thoughts are self-deprecating and, when this is extreme, it may lead to a cognitive / affective disorder such as depression or to a person becoming obsessive about certain aspects of their lives. We will look at this further in *Chapter 4*, when we use Transactional Analysis (TA) to explore internal dialogue, but there are other theories that can help us understand how thinking influences feelings and vice versa.

Cognitive Behavioural Therapy (CBT) as established by Arron Beck (1989) seeks to help the person change how they think and feel about themselves. Abramowitz (2001) suggests that CBT is a really effective technique that can be used in almost any setting. Developing such a skill may prove to be of interest to you as you progress through your studies but that detail is not explored any further here, other than to give you these references for further reading. Mindfulness-based cognitive therapy (MBCT), as mentioned previously, is another technique which helps us to alter our thoughts and feelings in positive ways. You can find out more about mindfulness and MBCT on the Mental Health Foundation's website, www.mentalhealth.org.uk.

What is evidenced in those texts and similar writings is that how we think and feel about ourselves impacts on our behaviour and consequently on how we communicate with the world. The more positive we are in our thoughts and perceptions of the world and ourselves, the more likely it is that we are more positive in our communications with others. Goleman (1996), in his book *Emotional Intelligence*, describes what he terms the 'Master Aptitude' in which he explores how personal narrative and self-talk influence us as human beings. If we believe we can do a thing, the likelihood is that we can. For Goleman 'hope' and 'optimism' are our great motivational forces and it is positive thinking that makes all the difference to our mood, our emotional sense of self, how we communicate, and our success.

For example, if we believe ourselves to be hopeless at speaking French we try to avoid speaking it and rely on others to communicate for us if the need arises. We would hold ourselves back from the conversation and push others ahead to do the talking. The thoughts that may go through our heads in that situation may include, 'I'm not good enough, my French teacher was always telling me my accent was atrocious, I will make a total fool of myself, best to leave it up to the others'.

The consequences of holding back may then be perceived by others involved in that communication as our being lazy, shy or just plain ignorant. It all depends upon the other person's interpretation of our avoidance behaviour. They may then throw us a look that results in us feeling even more inadequate and more negative about the situation and ourselves. It reinforces our negative thinking about how hopeless we actually are and it can tap into previous memories and similar experiences when we felt like this. Inevitably this leads to more negative thinking, which impacts further on our behaviour and may make us even more resistant to speaking French. We develop patterns of behaviour that initially seek to protect us but often result in an over-reaction to a given situation. Negative thinking often leads to poor performance which, in turn, is reinforced by ourselves and maybe even by others.

If we apply this example to a healthcare setting we can see how negative thinking can seriously impact on the way that we communicate with others. If someone has always been told they are as quiet as a mouse, not very sociable, lacking in confidence, they will inevitably think negatively about their ability to communicate in an easy and relaxed way with a patient in a hospital or a resident in a care home. They might avoid situations where they have to work one-to-one with someone, preferring to stay in the background. Their shyness might be construed as aloofness or rudeness and they may then find it more difficult to form positive relationships because colleagues and patients or residents avoid them. However, it is possible to reframe those descriptions:

| Negative | Positive |
|---|---|
| 'Quite as a mouse' | 'Good listener' |
| 'Not very sociable' | 'Good at one-to-one interaction' |
| 'Lacking in confidence' | 'Quietly assured' |

Viewed in that way, the person would feel very different about themselves and might interact with others in a different and very valuable way.

**REFLECTION** 2.4

Think of an example of negative thinking that has affected you.
- Can you think of another personal event or issue that you have that leads to this downward spiral of negative thinking?
- How does that impact on your behaviour?
- What is the outcome of that behaviour on you and on others?
- Can you think of ways in which you could change the outcome?
- What do you imagine the result would be?

We've all been in situations that we know we could have handled differently and where the outcome could have been more beneficial to all concerned if only we had gone about it in a different way. One of the techniques many people use to counteract these negative responses is self-talk. Using key words like 'steady', 'focus', 'stay with the moment', 'don't panic', 'think', 'breathe in slowly', 'take your time' are tools we often use to help us regulate our thoughts and behaviour. Changing the dialogue in your head is a good technique to avoid falling into patterns of behaviour and using positive thinking can cancel out the negative thoughts.

## POSITIVE THINKING

The power of positive thinking should never be underestimated. Positive thinking can enhance our performance enormously. Positive thinkers engage in positive internal dialogue that reinforces and affirms their competence and their ability to do well. We occasionally get to see or read about famous people and what they do to 'psych themselves up' before going on stage. That's the power of positive thinking – it changes our mind-set and results in different behaviour. If we think positively we will feel positive and it is then more than likely that we will act in a different way.

You may have techniques to get yourself through tricky situations. Warming up by clapping, thinking or even thinking the words 'come on, I can do this' are all examples of positive internal dialogue. As you 'warm up' you may even verbalise or portray some of those warming-up actions and share them with others. The result may be that you gain their support which, in turn, has the potential to improve your performance or at least your mind-set. In a situation where everyone is backing you, urging you on, clapping and offering their support you are encouraged and your behaviour will be changed or enhanced in some way. Developing the skill of reflection and examining your own internal thoughts and patterns of behaviour can help enormously.

## REFLECTION AND REFLECTIVE PRACTICE

Reflection involves looking back at events and asking questions and looking forward at possible outcomes and asking questions. Alsop and Ryan (1996) suggest that reflection is both retrospective and prospective.

Retrospective reflection is like looking at a photograph or a video. It tells us about ourselves in the past, where we were or what we were doing.

Prospective reflection is like looking at a holiday brochure or video before we go away. We get ideas of what it might be like, what we might do or whom we will meet. It is almost like superimposing ourselves into the picture.

Reflection is important because it helps us to learn and make sense of our experiences. "Reflection is an important human activity in which people recapture their experience, think about it, mull it over and evaluate it. It is this working with experience that is important in learning" (Boud *et al.*, 1985, p. 19). So, the key way of increasing our self-awareness is through reflection, either alone or with other people. Reflective practice is the application of the skill of reflection to our practice with the intention of improving our professional practice. It is a way of not only increasing our self-awareness but of helping us to make sense of our experiences in professional contexts.

Things go wrong for a multiplicity of reasons; we are not robots and we cannot be perfect. In fact, if we were perfect or even tried to be, it is unlikely that people would like us very much. We are all flawed, we have our blind spots, we have prejudices and sometimes we clash with other people and end up saying, doing or thinking things that are not helpful to us or those around us. The more curious, aware and open we are about when, why and how things go wrong, the more able we are to work ethically. Oelofsen (2012) suggests that being a reflective practitioner "involves developing a sophisticated understanding of the interplay between individual, systemic, and organisational factors, as well as developing a strong sense of the impact of your own dynamics on these processes" (p. xiii). He goes on to say that becoming a reflective practitioner involves a process of personal growth and an understanding of the assumptions (or values and beliefs) inherent in your own approach to practice.

A good starting point would be to reflect on your own strengths and weaknesses using a simple SWOT (Strengths, Weaknesses, Opportunities, Threats) analysis. *Figure 2.1* is an example which shows how this can help to focus on the areas of your interpersonal skills that are good and can be enhanced, and those that need development. It also encourages you to think about what helps and hinders you in communicating with others.

| STRENGTHS | WEAKNESSES |
|---|---|
| • Outwardly confident<br>• Chatty<br>• Friendly<br>• Interested in other people's stories<br>• Have plenty of experience of working with people | • Hide my lack of confidence in some situations by being too chatty<br>• Get emotional when I'm tired and hungry<br>• Lose my temper when I see someone being unfair<br>• Feel intimidated by people in authority |
| OPPORTUNITIES | THREATS |
| • Have good mentor who is friendly and approachable<br>• Have good relationships with my family and friends<br>• Have line manager meetings every week<br>• Have access to courses and training | • Work long shifts and get really tired<br>• Feel a bit scared of line manager who seems really unapproachable<br>• Don't really know what I'm doing sometimes and am worried I'll get caught out |

**Figure 2.1** *Example of a simple SWOT analysis.*

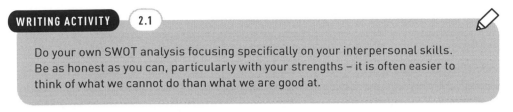

**WRITING ACTIVITY** 2.1

Do your own SWOT analysis focusing specifically on your interpersonal skills. Be as honest as you can, particularly with your strengths – it is often easier to think of what we cannot do than what we are good at.

Once you have reflected like this on your professional practice, you will find it easier to take the reflection a step further and think about specific situations where you feel changes need to be made.

## Reflective tools

A simple reflective tool which helps us to focus on specific situations and analyse what happened is Borton's Development Framework (Borton, 1970). This involves three simple steps:

**What** – happened, was I doing, were others doing? *Identify experience and describe detail.*

**So what** – more do I need to know to understand this, could I have done differently? *Analyse and interpret.*

**Now what** – do I need to do to make things better and what will be the consequences of my actions? *Explore alternatives and plan thoughtful action.*

Here is an example of how Borton's Development Framework can be used to reflect on an interaction in a workplace that went wrong:

**What?** Setting: A residential care home for the elderly. I was talking to the son of a resident, Mr C, about his father's low mood. The son was getting annoyed that his father wasn't being helped enough, that he was being left alone too often and that the staff should be giving him more stimulating activities to keep him busy. He seemed very anxious and a bit angry. This was the first time he'd been to see his father for three weeks and I snapped "Maybe if you came to see him a little more often, he'd be a bit happier". The son was really angry, shouted at me then complained to my manager.

**So what?** I realise that I spoke rudely to Mr C's son. I felt that he was being unfair because we make a lot of effort with the residents, especially his father because he has been feeling low and he's a really lovely man. I felt angry and annoyed with the son because he was blaming me and the rest of the staff when I think he should have been thinking about how he could help his father more. I know that I shouldn't have been so rude and that it's completely inappropriate to criticise the relatives of the residents but we've all been thinking the same thing for a while. When my grandad was still alive, we made sure that we looked after him in his own home and when he got too old and frail we moved him into our house so that we could look after him. It's hard for me to see people leave their parents in a home and not look after them themselves but I have to remember that not all families are the same as mine, we all do things differently and I shouldn't be so judgemental. I just can't help it!

**Now what?** I have to keep my thoughts to myself and not criticise the relatives of residents. I have to remember that not all people feel the same way that I do. If that situation arises again, I will make sure that I just listen to the complaints and say that I will do what I can to help. I will apologise to the son and I will make sure that I spend more time with Mr C.

This example shows that the worker has thought about the way that her values have impacted on the way that she interacted with the son of the resident and she understands that it was not professional. However, there are further opportunities for analysis and reflection if we use a different framework. If we want to take our reflections to a more detailed level we can use a number of other reflective tools which encourage us to analyse our practice in depth and to use our reflective skills, our self-awareness and our creativity to find alternative ways of approaching situations in professional contexts.

One of the most important skills to develop is curiosity. Reflective practice is based on the idea that as professionals we must always remain curious about what is happening, why it is happening and how we might make changes for the benefit of all. If we remain curious, we are more able to consider multiple ideas about a certain situation. We are also more able to avoid jumping to conclusions or making snap judgements, which might close down effective communication. In the situation described above, the worker's reflections could have gone deeper if she had been more curious about the son's situation, about his father's situation and about her response to them.

Oelofsen (2012) offers a useful framework called the Three-Step (CLT) Reflective Cycle (see *Figure 2.2*) which helps to structure our reflections and to remain curious about what might be happening. A simplified form of Kolb's (1984) Adult Learning Cycle, Oelofsen's CLT Reflective Cycle consists of the following three steps:

**Step 1: Curiosity**

This step involves noticing things, asking questions and questioning assumptions.

**Step 2: Looking closer**

This step involves looking at the situation in detail, finding words that help us to make sense of what has happened or what has been said. This stage must involve us being open to alternative perspectives and ideas, thinking about the situation from other positions and not falling back on accepted assumptions or methods.

## Step 3: Transformation and feedback

This step is about bringing together the thoughts and ideas from the previous two steps and finding ways of thinking about how a situation might be different and how positive changes can be made.

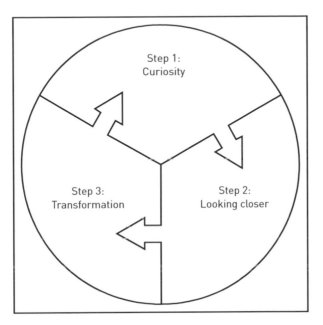

**Figure 2.2** *The three-stage (CLT) model of reflection.*

It is much easier to understand how to use a reflective tool like this when it is applied to an actual situation, so here is how we might use CLT to reflect on the scenario described above:

**Step 1: Curiosity**

I can't work out who I was more annoyed with after that altercation, Mr C's son who was having a go at me and this place or myself for losing my cool and being rude to him. I think that we all get a bit defensive when relatives criticise the work that we do here. We all work really hard and the care home has a very good reputation so it makes me mad when someone has a go. I wonder why we don't get used to it, it happens often enough. What should I do when I feel like I'm being criticised? I wonder why Mr C's son reacted that way. He hadn't been to see his father for 3 weeks, perhaps he's been away. He usually comes once a week and he's always been perfectly polite though not very chatty or friendly. He spends his time here talking about his work and his Dad always asks lots of questions. They seem to get on well though they aren't all that affectionate with each other, which is why I was so surprised that the son was so concerned about his Dad, he never seemed to be all that bothered before.

**Step 2: Looking closer**

Now that I think about it, I remember Mr C telling me that his son was a doctor, a surgeon in a hospital. He was really proud of that as he hadn't even been to University, I think he said that he had two grandchildren but he doesn't see them much as they live with their Mum. I think they've only been here once or twice and their Dad doesn't come here at the weekend because I think he goes to see the children. He must be really busy. Mr C has never complained about being here, he was happy to move in so I think he might have chosen to come and live here because he didn't want to get in the way of his son's job. Maybe he was really anxious about his Dad this time because he'd been away and hadn't seen him for 3 weeks – if that were me I'd feel really guilty. I think that when he was younger his Dad probably made loads of sacrifices for him so that he could go to medical school and now he's still putting him first by insisting that he lives here. He'd probably hate it if his son had to change his work in any way. The son has probably always felt a bit guilty that his Dad made those sacrifices for him and he hasn't been able to pay him back in the way he'd like. I'm beginning to understand his reaction to me a bit more now. Why did I have to snap at him like that? I guess that my family felt it was really important that Grandad lived with us, well, I know my Mum did and she didn't work full time so it was easier for her. Mind you, she did complain about him a lot when he got really grumpy. I think that it was ingrained in me that you have to look after your parents to the very end, however hard it got. My mum and dad will expect me to I'm sure – I hope that I won't need to! I really like Mr C, though he has got more grumpy and quiet in the last couple of months, just like my Grandad did. I guess he's not able to do the things he used to be able to do when he first got here, his joints are so sore and he gets dizzy when he stands. I'm finding it harder to keep him entertained and he doesn't follow what I'm saying the way he used to. It's probably the same when he talks to his son, he always wants to know how work is and asks him exactly what kind of procedures he has to perform and how he does it. I guess he's finding it more difficult to follow and that's frustrating for him. It must be really difficult for his son to see him like that, they always had such long and involved conversations.

**Step 3: Transformation and feedback**

I'm going to phone Mr C's son and apologise for being rude. I want to explain that the way I reacted to him was unfair as I was judging him without thinking about why he was feeling so anxious about his Dad. I am going to speak to my manager and tell her what I've been thinking. I want to discuss how our own experiences of looking after elderly relatives really impacts on the way that we see the relatives of our residents. We are quite judgemental sometimes and so I want us to do some training that will help us to reflect more on this. Maybe we should all try to have more discussions with each other about how we speak about residents and their relatives. We need to think more about why they might be behaving in certain ways or saying certain things. I think we tend to jump to conclusions too often. Next time I feel like I'm being criticised I need to take a breath and not act so defensively. It would have been so much better if I'd just said to Mr C's son "You seem really anxious about your Dad, shall we sit down and have a proper talk about what you feel he needs?"

As you can see, the CLT reflective model encourages you to reflect more deeply on the situation, being curious about what is going on and questioning assumptions so that you can gain insight into how your thoughts, values and beliefs have influenced the way that you communicate.

**WRITING ACTIVITY** **2.2**

Think of a situation where you feel that you weren't able to communicate effectively or where your interaction with someone else didn't go well. Use either Borton's Development Framework or the Three-Step CLT Reflective Cycle to explore and reflect on the situation and find alternative ways of approaching the same situation next time. It would be even more beneficial if you used first Borton, then the CLT model and see if the second one encourages you to be more curious and come up with more possibilities.

In an ideal situation, your work setting should be promoting reflective practice throughout the organisation, so that both managers and staff are constantly engaged in reflecting on how their practice can be developed and improved. If that is the case, you will be part of a team that encourages you to reflect on what you do, both by yourself, with your colleagues and with your managers. If it is not the case you should still be reflecting on your practice, using reflective tools and being curious so that you can develop your self-awareness and your skills.

**CHAPTER SUMMARY**

**Six key points to take away from Chapter 2:**

- Intrapersonal communication and self-awareness are essential interpersonal skills.
- The 'self' we choose to bring to our professional setting can affect the way that we communicate with our colleagues and the people in our care.
- We must be aware of how our physical and emotional state can affect the way that we communicate.
- We must know our limitations and recognise when we need help.
- Our values and beliefs can determine the attitudes we have and the way that we interpret and deal with situations and interactions.
- Reflective practice, both individually and with others, is an ideal way to improve your self-awareness and interpersonal skills.

## USEFUL READING

Cuthbert, S. and Quallington, J. (2008) *Values for Care Practice*. Exeter: Reflect Press.

Jasper, M. (2003) *Beginning Reflective Practice*. Cheltenham: Nelson Thornes.

Johns, C. (2004) *Becoming a Reflective Practitioner* 2nd ed. Oxford: Blackwell.

Oelofsen, N. (2012) *Developing Reflective Practice: A guide for students and practitioners of health and social care*. Banbury: Lantern Publishing.

## REFERENCES

Abramowitz, J.S. (2001) CBT for obsessive compulsive disorder; a review of the treatment literature. *Research and Social Work Practice*, **11(3):** 357–373.

Alsop, A. and Ryan, S. (1996) *Making the Most of Fieldwork Education: A practical approach*. Cheltenham: Stanley Thornes.

Association of American Medical Colleges (1999) Report III: *Contemporary Issues in Medicine*. Washington, DC: Communication in Medicine.

Beauchamp, T. and Childress, J. (2001) *Principles of Biomedical Ethics* 5th ed. New York: Oxford University Press.

Beck, A.T. (1989) *Cognitive Therapy and the Emotional Disorders*. London: Penguin.

Borton, T. (1970) *Reach, Teach and Touch*. London: McGraw Hill.

Boud, D., Keogh, R. and Walker, D. (1985) Promoting reflection in learning: a model. In D. Boud, R. Keogh and D. Walker (eds) *Reflection: turning experience into learning*. London: Kogan Page.

Cuthbert, S. and Quallington, J. (2008) *Values for Care Practice*. Exeter: Reflect Press.

Erikson, E. (1995) *Childhood and Society*. London: Vintage.

Goleman, D. (1996) *Emotional Intelligence. Why It Can Matter More Than IQ*. London: Bloomsbury.

Kabat-Zinn, J. (2004) *Wherever You Go, There You Are*. London: Piatkus.

Kolb, D. (1984) *Experiential Learning: Experience as the source of learning and development*. New Jersey: Prentice Hall.

Oelofsen, N. (2012) *Developing Reflective Practice: A guide for students and practitioners of health and social care*. Banbury: Lantern Publishing.

Rogers, C. (1961) *On Becoming a Person*. New York: Houghton Mifflin.

Vygotsky, L.S. (1966) Development of higher mental functions. In A.N. Leontyev, A.R. Luria and A. Smirnov (eds) *Psychological Research in the USSR*. Moscow: Progress Publishers.

# 03

# INTERPERSONAL COMMUNICATION

**KEY THEMES:**

- Interpersonal skills

- Verbal communication

- Non-verbal communication

- Environmental communication

- Intercultural communication.

In health and social care services, effective communication promotes the best possible care. It enables you to practise the highest possible standards of care and it can safeguard you in the case of legal or disciplinary action. The way we communicate with people who use our service or facility also has a direct impact on how care is perceived and experienced. More complaints are made about practitioners whose communication skills are poor than about professional expertise (Gladwell, 2005). Patient Advice and Liaison Services (PALS) annual reports, which are all available online, regularly detail staff attitude and poor communication skills as the main area of complaint.

**REFLECTION** — 3.1

"I remember a time when my baby daughter was seriously ill in hospital. The consultant paediatrician came to see her and immediately started looking at her chart without making eye contact or speaking either to her or to me. I started to talk to her and she brushed my questions away without even looking at me and spoke to one of the nurses. I was obviously very distressed and found it difficult to be assertive. I just wanted to cry and I felt small and unimportant and I have never forgotten it. There have been countless other occasions when I have experienced the warmth, respect and kindness of many other healthcare professionals."

Think about the times that you have been to hospital, been to your GP, spoken to any health or social care professional about either your own issues or those of someone you care about. What happened? What worked and what didn't work? How did the professional communicate with you?

# INTERPERSONAL SKILLS

If you have read through *Chapter 2*, done the activities and spent time reflecting on your values, beliefs and the way that you communicate these through your actions and attitudes, you will be in a good position to think about the communication that takes place between people and particularly between you and others. We refer to this as interpersonal communication and there are particular skills that are needed to ensure that we are communicating effectively in health and social care settings. The language we use, our non-verbal behaviours and the symbols we include in our interactions all play a powerful role in establishing and sharing meaning. As stated in *Chapter 1*, understanding of language and communication is a subjective experience, dependent on people's culture, age, gender and environment and the words that one person uses will be understood differently according to context. This chapter will encourage you to think about how we communicate both verbally and non-verbally, it will explore the ways that different environments affect communication and it will look at the implications of intercultural communication on health and social care workers and users.

Being competent in interpersonal communication is crucial for successful living and all communication theorists define interpersonal skills in a similar way. A skill is something that is seen as a motor activity that can be practised, developed and refined until perfection is achieved (Hargie, 1991). However, interpersonal skills are far more complex than that and involve a whole host of factors. Because the factors involved are so many, it is difficult to find a succinct academic definition that addresses all of these issues. Burnard (1989) commented that "what constitutes interpersonal skills is vast", and he goes on to suggest that "personal qualities are a necessary pre-requisite for effective interpersonal relationships". It is likely that you either work, or you are going to work, in areas that require you to have effective personal relationships with the people you work with. It is therefore essential that you develop and demonstrate these qualities. The personal qualities that Burnard (1989) alludes to are based on those of Carl Rogers (1951) and include "warmth and genuineness, empathic understanding and unconditional positive regard". As Burnard states, "it is these qualities that form the basis and the bedrock of all effective human relationships". These qualities underpin helping relationships and are further discussed in *Chapter 5*.

**WRITING ACTIVITY** 3.1

Make a list of all the interpersonal skills you know. The list may be divided into those interpersonal skills you have and those skills you wish to develop in the future and may be divided further into subcategories if you wish. It's your perception and understanding of what constitutes an interpersonal skill that counts.

Now discuss your list with another person who you feel will be able to give you valuable feedback about your skills and, perhaps, add to the overall list.

**WRITING ACTIVITY** 3.1 CONT'D

Write down your thoughts on how and where we develop interpersonal skills and follow this through by using an example of your own.

No doubt your list is a long one detailing all sorts of things ranging from assertiveness to values, attitude to understanding, empathy to questioning. You may have included clusters of communication skills such as verbal and non-verbal behaviours and it is likely that you have used some of the previous detail in responding to the second question.

If you have discussed this with someone you should have an insight into how skilled a person you already are and gained some insight into how you have developed those skills. We can usually say how and where our interpersonal skills have developed. Interpersonal skills are learned. They are learned through observation and practice, they are a result of previous experience and intrapersonal reflection and evaluation. Just as we learn our values and beliefs during childhood, we also learn interpersonal skills and we can continue to develop them throughout our lives.

Interpersonal skills are culture-bound, age-related and often gender specific. They reflect the sort of person we are. We often use interpersonal skills without thinking, as they are so ingrained within our behaviour. Through reflection and detailed analysis, alongside a desire to learn, we can develop and refine those skills. Becoming more competent at human communication will enable you to become more competent in your role of helping others. When analysing and evaluating our interpersonal skills it's vital to remember that face-to-face communication happens both verbally and non-verbally.

## VERBAL COMMUNICATION

Language, whether it be spoken or signed, is the vehicle for allowing us to express who we are and how we relate to those around us. Koprowska (2010, p. 12) suggests that "spoken messages are like a braid of which only one strand are the words themselves". Clearly, what we communicate non-verbally has a massive impact on the way that our message is received but the words that we use are vitally important too.

The old adage "sticks and stones may break my bones but words will never hurt me" is one that has been trotted out for decades to try to diminish the importance of people's hurtful and careless utterances, but I think that most of us would agree that words have indeed hurt us and they have certainly got us into trouble. I have never forgotten a PE report when I was a very tall, big-footed 13-year old that said I was a "very ungainly child". This stuck with me for years and certainly influenced the way that I thought about myself and my appearance. The words that we choose and the way that we say them have the potential to be devastating but they can also have a hugely beneficial impact on the people that we interact with, especially, as is often the case in professional settings, when we are working with people who might be vulnerable or going through a difficult transition in their lives. When we know someone well, we are usually in a position to qualify or correct or apologise for things that we might have said that have seemed careless or hurtful. In work settings, we might not know the people that we come across very well; first impressions are important and especially if they are relying on us for support, the way that we speak to them can make an enormous difference to how they feel.

The relationships that you will have with people in the work setting will often involve complex communication and so it is essential to remember that the context of the words spoken can depend on so many different things; the way they are said, where they are said, who says them and who hears them. Giving guidance on how to communicate verbally is difficult; effective communication is not an exact science and if we start to create rules about how to communicate we are in danger of taking away the natural, warm and genuine way that people communicate with those in their care. We are all different and where one person might find formal communication comforting and appropriate, another might find it cold and impersonal. This section gives you ideas to reflect on and encourages you to think about the way that you use verbal communication without being too prescriptive. Throughout this book you are asked to reflect on verbal communication in conjunction with other important elements but at this point, it would be useful to think about how we verbally initiate any interaction in a health and social care setting.

Language is subjective and people may attach different meanings to the same message depending on their experience, environment, age, gender, culture; even what might have happened to them five minutes ago. When considering the importance of verbal communication with people in health and social care settings we need to be aware of the impact of our choice of language on them. Words and phrases can have a denotative or surface meaning, and a connotative or hidden meaning. A seemingly harmless comment like "You look tired today" might have been intended as a mere statement of fact (denotative) but depending on the way it is said it could be construed as rude or sarcastic or critical (connotative). Moreover, the mood and mind-set of the person hearing the comment might decide that the speaker is saying "You look dreadful" or "You look old". A simple question like "How are you feeling today?" would avoid most possible pitfalls and allow the person being asked to say as much or as little as they want.

## First impressions

Most of us would agree that making snap judgements about people as soon as we meet them is not good practice in any setting but we must be honest and admit that many of us do. Making a good impression at the outset is an important ingredient in forming good relationships with the people that we care for. The way that we communicate verbally when we first meet someone will depend on the context and on the needs of the person that we are communicating with. Rather than give specific advice on what words to use, the following subheadings invite you to consider and reflect on how you might approach the first moments of meeting someone new.

## Greetings

"Hello" is likely to be the most commonly used greeting, followed by an introduction if we haven't met the person before. We will often go on to say "How are you?" or more formally "How do you do?" which is often more of a rhetorical question than a genuine desire to know how someone is. More informal greetings, ones like "Hi", "Hiya", "All right?" will depend on the context and environment. Some greetings will belong to a particular dialect or culture and be appropriate in some settings more than others. We are likely to adapt the way that we greet someone when they are better known to us.

It can be quite disconcerting when you meet someone new and they immediately start talking without the usual greetings like "Hello". "Hello" or "Hi" are like the capital letter at the beginning of a sentence, they signify to us that we have been seen and acknowledged or that a conversation is about to begin.

Think about the many different ways that we can say the simple word "Hello". The meaning of even this simple five-letter word can be altered depending on the context, the pitch, tone, volume, body language or even mood of the speaker and listener. Try saying it aloud in as many ways as you can – you will see how the meaning is changed each time.

**REFLECTION** 3.2

Take some time to notice how you and others say the word "Hello". When you are first greeted by someone in a formal setting, what greeting would you expect or want to hear? What does it feel like when someone says "Hello" in a flat voice and doesn't make eye contact with you? Do you tend to say "Hello" in different ways depending on the setting and the person that you are greeting?

## Names

Names are vitally important. Our name defines us, gives us our identity and individuality. I have an unusual surname so I am very used to people pronouncing it wrongly. I prefer it when people ask me how to pronounce it rather than assume they know. I find it really surprising that even when I tell them how to pronounce it, they continue to say it wrongly. I am equally surprised, and very pleased, when someone gets it right. I notice it immediately and feel more open to that person, probably because I feel as if they have taken an interest. I also like to know the name of the person that I am speaking to and will ask them if they haven't told me. The way that someone wishes to be addressed is a personal thing; some prefer first names, while some prefer titles and surnames. When I was a child, my friends always addressed my parents as Mr and Mrs Pavord but now I would find it very strange if my children's friends called me by my surname. When meeting women it can be more complicated because there are three possibilities; Miss, Ms or Mrs. When meeting parents we cannot assume they have the same surname as their children so it can be difficult to know what to call them. I have noticed that when my children have appointments, some professionals will refer to me as Mum when speaking directly to me which I find strange as I am obviously not their Mum so I will always say "my name is Erica".

In many situations we are already likely to know the name of the person that we are about to meet but we must not assume that they want to be addressed by their first name, or by their title and surname and so it is important to ask what they prefer to be called and then ensure that we continue to call them the name they have asked us to use. Simply asking the question "What do you like to be called?" indicates that you are interested in that person as an individual. Inevitably there are times when we might forget someone's name, especially when we meet a lot of new people and we don't see them regularly. In situations like these, the old adage "honesty is the best policy" applies. It's usually obvious when someone is trying to avoid saying your name and it can be far more off-putting than if you say "I'm so sorry, I've forgotten your name".

## Pet names

I am the youngest of four children and it's a long-standing joke in my family that our father calls all of us "darling", not so much through affection, but because he can't remember our names! Pet names can be a sign of affection and are often used within families and among friends. It is not uncommon for some people to use pet names as a matter of course with whoever they meet, for example "Love", "Darling", "Sweetheart" or less 'pet-like' names such as "Mate" and "Guv". People use them unconsciously and many don't question being called by them either, because they are often embedded in a culture and dialect. There are times, however, when people take offence or are irritated that their names are being ignored. They might feel that a certain intimacy is being assumed and prefer that a professional distance is maintained. As health and social care professionals we need to be able to read situations carefully and take the lead of the person we are speaking to. Initial introductions should be warm and formal at the same time. As the relationship develops, it might become more informal but this should be initiated by the service user rather than the professional.

## After the introductions

After the initial introductions it is likely that we will go on to ask questions about how someone is or to give them information. *Chapter 5* gives guidance on questioning and on active listening skills and verbal communication is covered further. Once the greeting and introductions have been made, we may not need to be interacting verbally because we are performing particular tasks and getting on with it quietly is more appropriate. Many people working in health and social care settings will have to be interacting with those in their care in quite an intimate way, helping them with washing, bathing, dressing and going to the toilet. Personal space is important to people but will need to be invaded if they are unable to perform basic physical tasks. This has the potential to be embarrassing and people may feel that their dignity is diminished. It is important to be respectful of this and to ensure that we are working in partnership with the service user, letting them know what we will be doing and asking them how they would prefer it is done. Your embarrassment will only increase theirs, so be open and straightforward. Sometimes there might be very little choice about how a task is performed or the person you are caring for is unable to talk, and in these situations it is equally important that you inform them what you are going to do and how you will do it.

**REFLECTION** 3.3

Take some time over the next few weeks to notice how people greet you and how they introduce themselves and address you. Think about your reaction to the way that you are addressed in different situations. If you are already working in a health and social care setting, notice how different people communicate verbally and reflect on what is more or less successful.

## Things to remember about verbal communication

- The words that we use to communicate are just one aspect of our communication but they are vitally important.
- The context of the words spoken can impact on their meaning; people may attach different meanings to the same message depending on the context.
- First impressions are important; on meeting, introduce yourself, saying your name and your role and ask how the person prefers to be addressed.
- Speak clearly and avoid jargon or technical language.
- Explain what it is you are going to do or what it is you need.
- Check that the person you are talking to has understood what you have said.
- Try to take your lead from the person that you are helping – if they are chatty and relaxed, talk back to them. If they make it clear that they don't want to chat,

don't fill the silences for the sake of it; keep things relevant to the task you are carrying out.

- The words that you choose depend on the way that you say them so ensure that your non-verbal communication matches your verbal communication.

## PARALANGUAGE

Paralanguage lies somewhere between verbal and non-verbal communication. It refers to the different way we moderate our speech through the pitch, tone, volume, rhythm and timing as well as ums and ahs, grunts and sighs. Hargie (2011, p. 81) says "How information is delivered paralinguistically has important consequences for how much of the message is understood, recalled and acted on". Sometimes the paralanguage fits well with the verbal language and the message is received more clearly. If we are trying to be assertive our tone and pace need to match our intention. It's difficult to sound assertive if our voice is really slow and relaxed or if it is fast and breathless. Awareness of what message our tone is communicating can help us to avoid difficult situations. Our words might be polite and appropriate but we sound bored and uninterested or, worse, rude and dismissive; this lack of awareness could make a huge difference to the success of the work you want to do and kind of support you need to give. Many people might choose not to return for subsequent appointments or might avoid talking about problems they have because they are put off or even intimidated by the way that the professional is speaking. Non-verbal encouragers like 'mmm', 'ahh', 'huh?' can be important, unintrusive ways of signifying that we are listening to someone, but if overused might signal that we are only pretending to listen. There are times when we use paralanguage inappropriately because we are trying to give the impression of listening when in fact we are busy writing lists in our head or thinking that we wish this person would just be quiet. I have been caught out like this when my children have been telling me long, convoluted tales and I say 'Ohh' in an excited way when I should have sounded sad or sympathetic!

It is equally important to be aware of the paralanguage of the people we are talking to. If there is a mismatch between the words spoken and the way they are spoken it can tell us a lot about the speaker's real meaning. We might be listening to someone who is talking about going home after a long stay in hospital. They say they are pleased to be leaving hospital and excited to finally be back at home but their tone is uncertain, their volume is quiet and their pace is hesitant. If we were to take what they say at face value, we might be ignoring the fact that they actually feel worried and a bit fearful. In situations like these it's important to notice the mismatch and allow the speaker an opportunity to say more about what they are feeling. They might decline the invitation to speak more openly but they might welcome the opportunity to talk about their concerns with someone understanding and supportive who can reassure them that their reticence is perfectly normal.

REFLECTION 3.4

Spend some time listening to the paralanguage that people use. Do they use a lot of 'umms'? Does it help or hinder the way that they communicate? When they are listening to one other person, do they use paralanguage to show that they are listening? Can you tell when someone is using paralanguage but they are definitely not listening? Try to notice how much paralanguage you use and think about whether it differs according to the situation.

## Things to remember about paralanguage

- The paralanguage that we use impacts on the message we convey.
- Our pace and tone and volume need to be appropriate to the situation and the message we want to convey.
- Show that you are listening through non-verbal encouragers but do not over-use them.
- It's important to be aware of the paralanguage of the person you are listening to and be aware of what it is communicating to you.

## NON-VERBAL COMMUNICATION

Professor Albert Mehrabian, a pioneer of communication research, suggested that 55 per cent of what is communicated is said to be communicated via body language, 38 per cent is communicated via voice tonality (sometimes referred to as paralanguage) and only 7 per cent of the communication relies on the actual words spoken (see *Figure 3.1*).

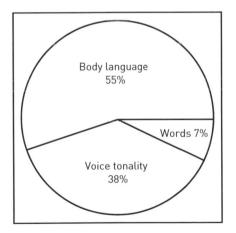

**Figure 3.1** *Mehrabian's Communication Model (1972).*

These statistics are often over-simplified and applied to all interactions but it is important to point out that his research findings apply specifically to spoken interactions which are emotional in content. This is particularly pertinent to communication in health and social care settings as so much of the communication is emotional in content and requires us to be alert to people's feelings and thoughts, concerns and fears.

In two separate studies looking at patients' perceptions of healthcare professionals' non-verbal communication (Chan (2012) and Marcinowicz *et al.* (2010)), it was found that those with better non-verbal communication skills have:
- better compliance
- better results
- better patient/client satisfaction
- fewer complaints.

Eye contact, posture/body language, facial expressions, gestures, interpersonal space, touch, smell, even clothes and general appearance are all important ways of communicating meaning. Think about the way that we are able to display emotions and attitudes through our non-verbal communication. We don't need to say anything for people to know we are excited, sad, bored or angry and often it is very difficult to hide these emotions even if we are saying that everything is fine.

**REFLECTION** 3.5

Spend some time over the next few days taking notice of people's non-verbal communication. Even if you can't hear what they are saying, you will probably be able to get a sense of the mood and purpose of their communication. Ask a trusted friend or family member to tell you what they notice about your non-verbal communication when you are talking to others.

Non-verbal communication supports and reinforces verbal communication and is essential if a message is to be conveyed with any conviction. If we tell someone we are happy, it will be accompanied by a smile and an upbeat tone. Conversely, non-verbal communication can complicate or contradict a verbal message. If we say we are happy but are frowning and our voice is tense and strained it is unlikely that anyone will be convinced. It is common for people in health and social care settings to want to give the impression that they are coping OK and that things are fine, because they don't want to take up the time of the busy professionals around them. Their non-verbal communication, if looked at closely, might give us a different picture if we took time to notice.

## Clothes and general appearance

In many jobs you are asked to wear a uniform, particularly jobs where effective hygiene and prevention of infection are of vital importance. Uniforms which are clean and smart are also important because they influence people's perceptions of the standards of care they experience. Uniforms give us a professional identity and allow people to easily identify who is in the care team. In some jobs uniforms are unnecessary but it is still important that we dress appropriately and think about the impression we are giving. As a counsellor I think that if I wore a uniform or a smart suit, I would give the wrong impression and it might affect the success of me building a therapeutic relationship, as I could be perceived as a distant and formal professional. Equally, if I wore clothes that were scruffy or overly casual like shorts and a strappy vest top I would be being overly informal and might communicate the message that I wasn't going to take my client all that seriously. Cleanliness and personal hygiene are vitally important. It's difficult to listen to someone, receive help or take advice from them if they are obviously unclean and smelly!

## Posture

The way that we stand or sit can communicate a lot about our mood and attitude and can show someone how ready we are to listen to them and communicate in a positive way. Ideally we should keep an open posture with uncrossed arms and legs but sometimes it feels more natural to keep our posture more matched to the person that we are speaking to. If we are standing whilst talking to someone and asking them if they need our help, it is important that our posture communicates a willingness to help by being open. If we stand with our arms crossed and our body angled away from the person, our words might be saying "Do you need help?" but our body is saying "I haven't got time or don't want to help you".

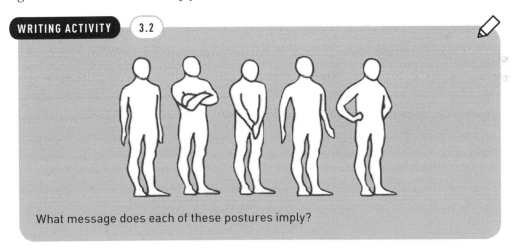

**WRITING ACTIVITY** 3.2

What message does each of these postures imply?

## Gestures

Some of us gesture more than others when we are talking and sometimes gestures can be engaging and animated. Gestures can be useful for emphasis although sometimes they can emphasise the wrong thing and give the wrong message. Gestures like finger tapping, looking at your watch, fidgeting, chewing your nails or playing with your hair can be distracting and off-putting.

## Facial expression

The main function of our facial expressions is to convey emotion and we are mostly unaware of what emotion we are displaying through our facial expressions until it's too late. Eckman (2007) suggests that there are six key emotions that people can discriminate, regardless of culture:

- Happiness/pleasure
- Fear
- Sadness
- Anger
- Surprise/shock
- Disgust.

For a patient in a hospital burns unit to see an expression of disgust on a nurse's face when he or she changes a dressing could have a devastating effect. Lightly veiled anger on the face of a care worker can be frightening for an elderly dementia patient. A smiling and happy looking face would be inappropriate if the patient is talking about their difficulties or if delivering bad news.

It is often best to keep a neutral expression on your face unless it is obvious that smiling is appropriate. As a counsellor I have to be very aware of what my face is communicating as I spend so much time listening to people's stories. I have often been told by clients that they were reluctant to come to counselling because they thought the counsellor would be some kind of 'do-gooder' with their head tilted to one side and a sickly and sympathetic smile on their face. Thankfully no one has accused me of that when they have actually come to see me.

## Eye contact

Eye contact is an important component of human behaviour and will be written about further in the body language section of *Chapter 5*. We tend to notice when someone either prolongs or avoids eye contact. If we maintain eye contact for too long it can be intimidating, confrontational or too intimate, depending on the context. Lack of eye contact can lead people to feeling ignored or excluded. We normally maintain eye contact for the duration of a conversation but break it for seconds at a time by looking away without moving our heads. The level of eye contact people are comfortable with can vary but in health and social care settings, professionals should ensure that they make eye contact with the person they are communicating with as much as possible to show that they are available and willing to listen.

## Touch

Often touch is an inevitable and vital part of your communication with people in health and social care settings, particularly when they need physical support with everyday tasks, and in cases like this touch should be appropriate to the task. When communication does not involve physical contact it can be confusing to know whether touching someone feels appropriate or not, especially when you are with someone in distress. During secondary teacher training, many years ago, I was told very firmly; "Never touch in praise nor anger". This seemed reasonable and unequivocal but in reality, to people who are naturally tactile, it can feel very unnatural not to comfort someone in distress by touching them, holding their hand, putting your hand on their shoulder or hugging them.

Touch can be caring and reassuring, it can express emotion and sometimes this can be useful or detrimental to the relationship. On the other hand, touching can be frightening, depending on the person's own history. It can seem like sensory overload for some and feel too intimate and even invasive.

Often certain settings will have guidelines and policies about touching and this will be to safeguard both worker and service user/client. In the literature of counselling and psychotherapy the therapeutic advantages or disadvantages of touching are debated at length. In general, touching is not advised as even when someone is very upset, touching them as a way of comfort can, inadvertently, communicate that you are not able to bear their distress. It is quite common for the listener to reach out to comfort the person in distress by touching them at the same time as saying "It's OK, don't cry". Although meant as comforting, this could be heard as, "Don't be sad, I can't handle your sadness". The physical touching acts as a brake to the conversation, halting the person's need to express their sadness. Remaining physically close, keeping eye contact and being completely present for the person in distress is often a better way to show support.

# ENVIRONMENTAL COMMUNICATION

Think about the way health and social care providers communicate with people who use their services. It might be helpful to walk around your workplace and observe the means of communication used there, or walk around a service facility that is open to the public or one that you would use. Make a mental note of what you see around you and consider the essence of the communications you observed.

1.  How would you describe these communications?
2.  What form do they take and how do they make you feel?

To explore this further think about a visit to your local GP surgery or health centre. In an average GP surgery or health centre you will be able to observe and experience many different formats of communication, including most of the following.

- To get an appointment with anyone who works at the health centre it is likely that you will have to telephone first. This may involve you being placed in a telephone queue, pressing appropriate telephone keys in response to pre-recorded instructions and it may take a little time.
- You will have to converse with a receptionist (fingers crossed that he or she can understand your use of verbal language, accent, dialect, etc.) and negotiate your appointment in relation to the urgency of your request and the person whom you would most like to see or deal with.
- When you arrive at the centre there are lots of directional instructions regarding where you can park (your car or your pushchair), where you should enter the building and that 'children should be under supervision'.
- As you enter the building there will be lots of healthcare / promotional posters on the walls. These are usually instructional and involve detail about the dangers or benefits of several everyday activities such as smoking, drinking alcohol and drug abuse. Magazines and health information leaflets are also likely to be available for your perusal.
- A zero tolerance poster stating that aggressive or rude behaviour will not be tolerated is now common in health centres, as are signs that say all mobile phones should be turned off. There will also be some signage about health and safety, in particular about fire assembly points, and signs directing you to toilet facilities.
- There may be a television screen that flashes up messages regarding services available at the health centre and promoting flu jabs, etc. and it may tell you how many people missed their appointment last week.
- There may be a touch screen on which you can key in your arrival and confirm your appointment and there may be signage telling you that if you are waiting to see a certain person they have a trainee working with them and that, with your permission, the appointment will be recorded.
- There may be a bell or light system indicating when you should enter the consulting room or you may have to wait on the nod of the receptionist. The person that you have come to see may shout your name down the corridor or even come and collect you from the waiting area.
- You might find yourself offered the opportunity to complete a questionnaire about your experience and satisfaction with the service.
- Lots of this detail will be presented in different languages that represent those spoken in the local community.

All this and you don't feel very well … The health centre used in this example sounds like a newly-built facility. It is bright and freshly painted and the communications are all up-to-date. The receptionists are most helpful and look very smart in their new uniforms. There is a notice advising that email requests for repeat prescriptions are accepted and that there is a prescription collection and delivery service offered via local pharmacies. Feelings about this kind of health centre are generally positive, although sometimes the amount of instructional material can be a little overwhelming (but it can give us something to do while waiting for the appointment). Some of the messages displayed will have an impact on our immediate behaviour so, for example, if your mobile phone rings you are likely to turn it off quickly, but many of the messages are part of a much bigger campaign to get health messages across to the general public and on their own they are often ignored.

However, sadly, we do have experiences of visiting other health care organisations where the facilities are lacking, the receptionists are rude, the décor is drab, toilets are dirty and information available is not up-to-date. All of this has an impact upon us as users of the service and we are more likely to be unhappy about our consultation even before we meet the professional we have booked to see.

**REFLECTION** **3.6**

The environment plays a big part in how we view services available to us. When you go back to your place of work or when you start work in a new environment what does the setting say about your service?

If your perception is negative, how do you think service users view the service?

How does the environment impact on the people who work there and the people who use the service?

## Things to remember about non-verbal language
- Non-verbal language communicates as much, if not more than verbal language.
- Dress appropriately and be aware of personal hygiene.
- Be aware of your posture, facial expression and the gestures you use when talking to someone as they can be off-putting and convey a negative message.
- Make eye contact with the person you are speaking to.
- Touch must be appropriate and relevant to the task you are carrying out.

# INTERCULTURAL COMMUNICATION

Britain in the 21st century is a culturally rich and diverse society, and health and social care services have to respond to the needs of this society through practices which both value the diversity and address the linguistic and cultural needs of the population. In order to understand how to do this we need first to understand what is meant by 'culture'. Our cultural identity is based not simply on our heritage but on our individual circumstances and our personal choice (Association of American Medical Colleges, 1999). Factors such as our gender, age, ethnicity, language, country of origin and acculturation; our sexual orientation, socio-economic status, religious or spiritual belief, our physical abilities and our occupation affect our sense of cultural identity. All of these factors may impact on our values and beliefs, our behaviour and lifestyle, our ways of communicating and our ways of understanding and interpreting the communication of others. The same words can mean different things to people from different cultures even when they speak the same language. When the language is different as well as the culture, the potential for misunderstanding is greater.

We all know that our words can be misunderstood, sometimes because we are using words that the other person does not understand. Sometimes the words are right but another part of our communication is misunderstood. The meaning that underlies our voice tonality, our body language and our words can all be misinterpreted. Cultural differences affect even simple gestures and because we communicate using symbols, social differences, even within the same culture, can affect communication. Most of the symbols we use during communication are learned when we are young and, therefore, some communication is not just culturally specific, it can also be specific to a family because you learn your basic communication symbols from your family. For one person the symbolic meaning of an extended period of eye-to-eye contact might mean that you are interested in what they have to say, while for another it could mean that you are being aggressive or threatening towards them.

It is important to be aware of how different cultures might interpret spoken language and body language. There are some non-verbal behaviours that are universal, like smiling, laughing and frowning but different cultures have different non-verbal languages as well as verbal ones. Ting-Toomey (1999) suggests that culture interferes with effective cross-cultural understanding in the following ways:

**Cognitive constraints:** different cultures have different frames of reference or world views that provide a particular lens through which all new information is seen.

**Behaviour constraints:** each culture has its own rules about behaviour which affects verbal and non-verbal communication.

**Emotional constraints:** different cultures regulate the display of emotion differently.

Sometimes, the obvious differences in culture are more straightforward than the less obvious. We are likely to be alert to the potential difficulties in communicating with someone from an obviously different culture from our own whose language, dialect or accent force us to listen and explain things more carefully. If the health and social care worker is from a different ethnic background from the ethnic majority in the UK, he or she is likely to be well aware of these potential difficulties and will probably have experience of dealing with people's attitudes and differing values.

More difficulties might arise when we assume that someone is from a similar culture to our own and we make a mistake or cause offence and a breakdown in communication occurs. "We need to question the invisible as well as the visible difference as the obvious dissimilarity is easier to take into account than the assumed equality" (Halson, 2005).

The image of an iceberg is a useful one to visualise when thinking about intercultural communication. Each culture has visible characteristics which impact on the way people from that culture are perceived: language, dress, food, music, physical appearance. Each culture also has invisible differences that impact just as much, if not more, on how meaning is made and how people interact with others: religious beliefs, rules, attitudes, views on raising children and caring for the ill and elderly, views on loyalty and friendship, the importance of time, education, gender roles and many more.

When differences in culture are obvious we need to be wary of times when we have preconceived ideas and assumptions about that culture because of stereotyped views. Stereotypes can be offensive because they are based on a generalised view of a group of people. They often single out a particular characteristic which might be shared by people of the same culture but they ignore the individuality of each person. In order to work ethically and communicate effectively we need to remember that each person is unique, a mixture of characteristics and qualities, and we have to attempt to understand each person from their own unique frame of reference (Ridley, 2005).

A useful model for helping us to raise our awareness of how cultural differences might impact on our communication comes from the world of Systemic Family Therapy. Burnham *et al.* (2008) developed the following acronym called the 'Social Grraacceess' to assist professionals working with families, reminding them to keep in mind the issues surrounding diversity and how they can affect the therapeutic relationship.

Gender

Race

Religion

Age

Ability

Class

Culture

Ethnicity

Education

Sexuality

Spirituality

They remind us that within the relationships that we form with clients, patients or service users there are differences that are one of the following:

**Visible and voiced** – this is when it is clear what the differences are and they are spoken about openly. It is in situations like these where the potential for misunderstanding is less likely, and when it happens it is noticed and can be dealt with.

**Visible and unvoiced** – this is when the differences are clear but they aren't spoken about, so when misunderstandings happen it is more difficult to be open and honest about how the communication has been affected. In situations like this, it is easy to see why one person might believe the other has acted in a prejudiced or discriminatory way.

**Invisible and voiced** – this is when the difference is not obvious but it is spoken about and brought into the open so again, there is less potential for misunderstanding.

**Invisible and unvoiced** – this is when differences are neither obvious nor spoken about. In situations like this it might be far more difficult to understand why communication has been difficult and more difficult to reflect on the reasons for it.

This is not, by any means, a suggestion that we should all be open about our differences in our professional contexts. That is a matter of personal choice and sometimes it might not be professional to disclose information if it is not relevant. It is simply a way of helping us to be curious about the cultural differences that may or may not be impacting on the way that we communicate with other people and to avoid making assumptions about what we think another person might be thinking and feeling.

**REFLECTION 3.7**

Think about the following scenario and decide which differences are:

Visible and voiced

Visible and unvoiced

Invisible and voiced

Invisible and unvoiced

A young British Black Caribbean male student nurse is helping an elderly man from Zimbabwe who is also black. He has recently arrived in the UK to visit his son and family and has been admitted to hospital following a fall and injury to his hip. The student nurse is in his final year and has been in a civil partnership for the last two years. He is wearing a wedding ring and speaks about his 'partner'. The elderly man was a Professor at the University in Harare and had close links with Robert Mugabe's government before he retired. Both nurse and patient are practising Christians.

Now that you have decided what the visible, voiced, invisible and unvoiced issues of diversity are or might be, reflect on the possible thoughts and feelings that each person in this interaction might have, depending on what they know and don't know.

This scenario will have shown you the many ways that our culture and the differences between us can impact on the way that we view and understand others. Whether differences were spoken about or not, there are likely to have been tensions in this scenario. The elderly man might have assumed the nurse was heterosexual. He might have had views about the nurse's job and level of education. The nurse might have seen his patient's age and acted in a certain way towards him or he might have assumed that he was vehemently homophobic, given his links to the Mugabe government which bans homosexuality. Their shared belief in Christianity might have implied a similarity which might or might not be there. The historical and cultural differences between Black African and British Black Caribbean are clear but someone who is only looking at skin colour might not take this into account. There are a multitude of factors which might impact on our communication as health and social care workers and it is our responsibility to be aware of them and ensure that they do not become barriers.

## Language barriers

When the differences in culture include language barriers, the potential for problems arising is greater.

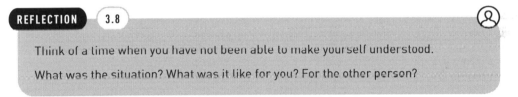

REFLECTION    3.8

Think of a time when you have not been able to make yourself understood.

What was the situation? What was it like for you? For the other person?

It is possible that you have thought of some or all of the following words to describe the feelings you might have had:
- Frustrated
- Unskilled
- Powerless
- Helpless
- Angry
- Embarrassed
- Loss of identity.

If we add that to the feelings already experienced by someone in a health and social care setting who needs support or advice or information, we can see that the language barrier brings with it huge pressure and stress, particularly for the person seeking help. Our cultural identity is inextricably linked to our language; we learn about our culture through language and our culture is transmitted through our language. In a situation where we are not able to express ourselves or make ourselves understood, we risk losing our sense of self and this can have a damaging impact on our self-esteem and self-worth. According to the 2011 Census carried out by the Office for National Statistics (2013):
- English is a second language to one in thirteen; more than 100 dialects are spoken by large numbers of people in the UK
- In England and Wales, 138 000 people cannot speak English at all

- More than 4 million people speak English as a second language – 7.7 per cent of the population
- Polish is the second most spoken language in the UK with 546 000 reporting it as their main language.

These statistics highlight the importance of providing high-quality interpreting services to all health and social care services to enable effective communication between the patient/service user and health and social care staff. The Equality Act (HMSO, 2010) states that all people should have equitable access to services, regardless of ethnicity or language spoken.

**REFLECTION** 3.9

You are a nurse working in outpatients and you are just about to meet a new patient, an asylum seeker from Syria called Dr F. You are told that an interpreter has been booked.

What are your thoughts and feelings?

What might Dr F be thinking about your appointment?

Some of the concerns might include:
- Is the interpreter going to be skilled enough to interpret accurately and will he or she speak the same dialect?
- Can I trust the interpreter to keep what he or she hears confidential?
- What religion or political ideology will the interpreter hold?
- Will the interpreter be sufficiently respectful?
- Will I feel ashamed or embarrassed, will I feel judged?
- If I need to come back again, will the same interpreter be used?

Tribe (2007) gives the following guidelines for professionals who need to use an interpreter:
- Create an atmosphere where each member of the triad feels able to ask for clarification and explanation when necessary
- Speak directly to the service user
- Minimise the use of specialist or technical language
- Use an interpreter who has experience of (and ideally training in) working within your area of expertise
- Consider the seating arrangements – an equilateral triangle usually works best
- Remember that you hold clinical responsibility for the meeting and explain this clearly
- Try to speak slowly and clearly and in short segments, because the interpreter has to remember what you have said and then interpret it

- Try to find someone from the same country. Matching for gender, age and religion may be useful, although this needs careful consideration
- Do not use a relative.

The last point is very important as very often family members or friends will be used as an interpreter, either at the request of the service user, or because it is the only option, especially in emergency situations. However, there are very important safeguarding implications when a family member or friend is used, particularly when the service user is vulnerable. The following is taken from the Serious Case Review of Daniel Pelka which pointed out the consequences of Daniel's older sister being used as an interpreter:

"Sometimes family members or the male partner was asked to act as interpreter, and whilst their use, particularly at times of an emergency or when a crisis situation arose was a pragmatic and understandable way to deal with a situation, overall it should have been balanced with opportunities to discuss the presenting situation in a more controlled and calm setting with an interpreter. Working Together states that 'Family members or friends should not be used as interpreters, since the majority of domestic and child abuse is perpetrated by family members or adults known to the child'." (Coventry Local Safeguarding Children Board, 2013).

# COMMUNICATING WITH THE DEAF OR PEOPLE WITH HEARING LOSS

There are a range of methods of communication for deaf people or those with hearing loss.
- Some will use sign language such as sign supported English or British Sign Language
- Lip reading and spoken English
- Note takers
- Speech to text reporters
- Electronic note takers

Communicating with someone who is deaf requires some thought and patience but it doesn't have to be complicated. Action on Hearing Loss (2014) provides the following useful guidelines for communicating with deaf people:
- Even if someone is wearing hearing aids it doesn't mean they can hear you perfectly. Ask if they need to lip read.
- If you are using communication support, always remember to talk directly to the person you are communicating with, not the interpreter.
- Make sure you have face-to-face contact with the person you are talking to.
- Get the listener's attention before you start speaking, maybe by waving or tapping them on the arm.

- Speak clearly but not too slowly, and don't exaggerate your lip movements – this can make it harder to lip read.
- Use natural facial expressions and gestures.
- If you're talking to a group that includes deaf and hearing people, don't just focus on the hearing people.
- Don't shout. It can be uncomfortable for hearing aid users and it looks aggressive.
- If someone doesn't understand what you've said, don't keep repeating it, try saying it in a different way instead.
- Find a suitable place to talk, with good lighting and away from noise and distractions.
- Check that the person you're talking to is following you during the conversation. Use plain language and don't waffle. Avoid jargon and unfamiliar abbreviations.
- To make it easy to lip read, don't cover your mouth with your hands or clothing.

**CHAPTER SUMMARY**

### Nine key points to take away from Chapter 3:

- Interpersonal communication is the communication that takes place between people and interpersonal skills are what we need to communicate effectively.
- The understanding of language, both verbal and non-verbal, is a subjective experience, dependent on context.
- When considering the importance of verbal communication with people in health and social care settings we need to be aware of the impact of our choice of language on them.
- Non-verbal communication such as clothes and general appearance, eye contact, posture/body language, facial expressions, gestures, interpersonal space, touch and smell, are all important ways of communicating meaning.
- The environment communicates directly to people in health and social care settings and can have an impact on the way that we communicate with those within that environment.
- Britain is a culturally rich and diverse society and health and social care services have to respond to the needs of this society through practices which both value the diversity and address the linguistic and cultural needs of the population.
- Cultural differences have an impact on communication. It is important to be aware of how different cultures might interpret spoken language and body language.
- In order to work ethically and communicate effectively, we need to avoid stereotypes and remember that each person is a unique individual.
- We need to work in partnership with interpreters to ensure that every person has equal access to services, regardless of ethnicity or language spoken.

## USEFUL READING

Baldwin, J., Means Coleman, R., Gonzalez, A. and Shenoy-Packer, S. (2014) *Intercultural Communication for Everyday Life*. Oxford: Wiley Blackwell.

Burnard, P. (1989) *Teaching Interpersonal Skills: A handbook of experiential learning for health professionals*. London: Chapman and Hall.

Koprowska, J. (2010) *Communication and Interpersonal Skills in Social Work* 3rd ed. Exeter, Learning Matters (*Chapter 3*: Human face of social work: emotional communication).

Moss, B. (2012) *Communication Skills in Health and Social Care* 2nd ed. London: Sage.

## REFERENCES

Action on Hearing Loss (2014). Communication tips. Available at: www.actiononhearingloss.org.uk/your-hearing/ways-of-communicating/communication-tips/tips-for-hearing-people.aspx (accessed 5 February 2015).

Association of American Medical Colleges (1999) Report III: *Contemporary Issues in Medicine*. Washington, DC: Communication in Medicine.

Burnard, P. (1989) *Teaching Interpersonal Skills. A handbook of experiential learning for health professionals*. London: Chapman and Hall.

Burnham, J., Palma, D. and Whitehouse, L. (2008) Learning as a context for differences and differences as a context for learning. *Journal of Family Therapy*, **30**: 529–542.

Chan, Z. (2012) A qualitative study on non-verbal sensitivity in nursing students. *Journal of Clinical Nursing*, **22**: 1941–1950.

Coventry Local Safeguarding Children Board (2013) Serious Case Review Re: Daniel Pelka. Available at: www.coventrylscb.org.uk/files/SCR/FINAL%20Overview%20Report%20%20DP%20130913%20Publication%20version.pdf (accessed 13 February 2015).

Eckman, P. (2007) *Emotions Revealed* 2nd ed. New York: Owl Books.

Gladwell, M. (2005) *Blink. The power of thinking without thinking*. Washington: Time Warner Books.

Halson, A. (2005) White – British or not. *Context*, **80**: 35–36.

Hargie, O. (ed.) (1991) *A Handbook of Communication Skills*. London: Routledge.

Hargie, O. (2011) *Skilled Interpersonal Communication. Research theory and practice* 5th edn. London: Routledge.

HMSO (2010) *Equality Act*. London: The Stationery Office. Available at: www.legislation.gov.uk/ukpga/2010/15/contents (accessed 13 February 2015).

Koprowska, J. (2010) *Communication and Interpersonal Skills in Social Work* 3rd ed. Exeter, Learning Matters (*Chapter 3*: Human face of social work: emotional communication).

Marcinowicz, L., Konstantynowicz, J. and Godlewski, C. (2010) Patients' perceptions of GP non-verbal communication: a qualitative study. *British Journal of Medical Practice*, **60(571):** 83–87.

Mehrabian, A. (1972) *Silent Messages: Implicit communication of emotions and attitudes.* Belmont, CA: Wadsworth Publishing.

Office for National Statistics (2013) *Language in England and Wales, 2011*. Available at: www.ons.gov.uk/ons/rel/census/2011-census-analysis/language-in-england-and-wales-2011/rpt---language-in-england-and-wales--2011.html (accessed 5 February 2015).

Rogers, C. (1951) The necessary and sufficient conditions for therapeutic change. *Journal of Consulting Psychology*, **21:** 95–103.

Ridley, C. (2005) *Overcoming Unintentional Racism in Counselling and Therapy* 2nd ed. London: Sage.

Ting-Toomey, S. (1999) *Communicating Across Cultures*. New York: Guilford Press.

Tribe, R. (2007) Working with interpreters. *The Psychologist*, **20:** 159–161. Available at: http://thepsychologist.bps.org.uk/volume-20/edition-3/asylum-4-working-interpreters (accessed 13 February 2015).

# 04

# INTRODUCING TRANSACTIONAL ANALYSIS

**KEY THEMES:**

This chapter introduces Transactional Analysis and explores:

- what Transactional Analysis is
- the concept of ego states
- the Parent ego state
- the Adult ego state
- the Child ego state
- transactions and analysing communication
- life scripts
- I'm OK, You're OK.

## WHAT IS TRANSACTIONAL ANALYSIS?

Transactional Analysis (TA) is a way of describing in a simple format that is easily understood what takes place within people and between people. It is a way of studying and making sense of intrapersonal and interpersonal relationships. It has at its core the belief that face-to-face communication is at the centre of human relationships, and if you are studying to develop your role in helping others it makes sense to include an overview of this theory in this book. What is offered here is my personal account of the work of Eric Berne, who was the originator of Transactional Analysis, and the work of other TA practitioners.

Eric Berne (1910–70) trained as a psychoanalyst and developed many theories during his lifetime. His work included six books (listed in the References) and he wrote many articles and edited the journal *Transactional Analysis Bulletin* until his death. He was the original founder of the International Transactional Analysis Association (TAA), which is the recognised professional body for therapists who use TA techniques in their psychotherapeutic work. TA is very popular in the USA and was popular in the UK during the 1960s and 70s. It is pleasing to see that it is again becoming popular, not only as a therapeutic technique but as a method for improving communications in organisations. You can study short courses on TA all over the country and some universities offer Masters-level degrees and doctorate programmes of study. For me, the work of Eric Berne removed the mystery that surrounds psychotherapy. Semenoff (cited in Klein, 1980) comments that "what Berne proposed was essentially Freud without the unconscious". TA uses everyday language resulting in an understandable theory that can be used by anyone as a method for understanding human communication and relationships.

## THE CONCEPT OF EGO STATES

At the heart of TA is the notion that our personality is made up of three alter ego states. Berne (1961) called these ego states **Parent, Adult** and **Child** (PAC). These terms have specific definitions within this theory and care should be taken to avoid misinterpretation with the everyday terms of parent, adult and child. Each ego state is said to have different qualities and different patterns of behaviour and, to be a fully functioning person, we need to have access to all of our ego states.

**The Parent ego state** is said to develop in us as children via the messages (teaching) we receive. It contains a great deal of recorded material that plays back and directs our behaviour. It is everything that we were taught.

**The Adult ego state** can be described as the thinking part of the self. It stores facts and processes information generated from within ourselves and from the external environment. It is everything that is thought.

**The Child ego state** holds all of the feelings that we have experienced in our lives, from anxiety to anger, depression to despair, happiness and joy. It holds all our fun and laughter. It is everything that is felt.

This simple model of a personality can provide us with an incredibly powerful tool to analyse our own and others' behaviour. You can spot which ego state someone is operating from, simply by the words that they use, their tone of voice and their gestures and behaviour. Analysing ego states is referred to as Structural Analysis and analysing transactions, i.e. those interactions that take place between people, is referred to as Transactional Analysis which we shall explore later. Let's move on and give you an opportunity to see if you can spot ego state characteristics and determine which is which. The details that follow are by no means comprehensive but they do give you an idea of how to spot which ego state you are accessing either in your own head or observing in others.

## The Parent ego state

The Parent ego state is full of moral messages stored as recordings and it has set patterns of behaving. Just like a parent it can be loving and doting and succour us throughout our lives. The Parent ego state can nurture and protect the self and others that it communicates with and has relationships with, but it can also spoil us by being over-indulgent. It can be controlling and help maintain order but it can also be condemning, critical and harsh. The Parent ego state within us reflects the qualities of those people who cared for us as small children. It will include parents and other people who acted as care givers such as grandparents, aunts and uncles, teachers, ministers of religion and people you admired and adored.

---

**REFLECTION** 4.1

Take some time to consider some of the people who were important to you in your life when you were a small child.

Can you recall any of the things that they regularly said?

What were the underlying messages behind the things that they said?

Do you live by those messages now?

---

I am happy to share one of my messages with you. My mother always used to say "no matter how hard it is, you've just got to get on with it". I live by that message now. There have been times in my life when things have been incredibly difficult but, guess what, no matter how difficult it has been I just "dust myself down" (another one of her sayings) and get on with it. My mother was, in the main, a very controlling parent; perhaps she needed to be with six children. I believe her mother was very controlling too, but I always knew I was loved and that she would sort things out for me if I got into difficulty. Please don't think that I had a perfect childhood as I didn't and I don't believe that a perfect childhood exists. In contrast to that supportive controlling way that she had, there were times when she was incredibly critical and patronising, but using TA as a framework to analyse her behaviour and my responses to it have enabled me to understand what took place between us and that insight into my own behaviour has enabled me to make alternative choices in the parenting of my own children.

What about you? It is likely that the things you value now are very similar to the things those people who were around you when you were small held dear. How often do you find yourself behaving in ways or saying the things that people did or said to you when you were small? I sometimes open my mouth and my mother's words spill out. My reaction is 'goodness, who invited mother into the conversation?' Now that I have that insight into my own behaviour I can choose to be like her or not, as the case may be. With that insight I now have the opportunity to change. Personal reflection on your own internal dialogues and examining where they came from and what they mean to you can enable you to develop your communication and relationship skills with others.

**WRITING ACTIVITY** ( 4.1 )

Using the simple framework provided here, detail what you would identify as the characteristics of the Parent ego state.

| Characteristics | Nurturing/Spoiling Parent | Controlling/Critical Parent |
|---|---|---|
| Words used | | |
| Tone of voice | | |
| Behaviours | | |
| Attitude | | |

### Parent ego state words

The Parent ego state uses phrases like: 'you must', 'you mustn't', 'you should', 'you shouldn't', 'you ought', 'you ought not', 'that's good', 'good boy', 'good girl', 'bad boy', 'bad girl', 'that's bad', 'just get on', 'just leave it', 'that's right', 'that's wrong', 'don't do this', 'don't do that', 'do this', 'do that', 'never mind', 'hurry up', 'stop that', 'mummy will do that', 'well done darling' and so on.

### Tone of voice

The Parent ego state uses two main tones, that of concern and that of authority. The voice can be either soft or loud, patronising or helpful.

Have you heard irate parents in the supermarket speak to their children through clenched teeth? They are incensed but they are saving the admonishment until the child is at home and away from the public eye. The tone can often suggest a different communication from the words used.

### Behaviours

The Parent ego state is also identifiable by its behaviours. Gestures, smiles, frowns, folded arms, open arms, pointing fingers, raised eyebrow, etc. are all markers of a Parent ego state.

### Attitude

The attitude displayed by a Parent ego state is what makes the whole communication tie together, or not, as the case may be. It can be giving and caring or moralistic, patronising and judgemental. It can be authoritarian and controlling or facilitating and helpful. The ego state's attitude is reflected in the words, tone, behaviour and other subtle paralanguage used within the communication and the relationship.

## The Adult ego state

**WRITING ACTIVITY** 4.2

Use the same process as in *Writing activity 4.1* and identify the characteristics of the Adult ego state.

| Characteristics | Adult ego state |
|-----------------|-----------------|
| Words used | |
| Tone of voice | |
| Behaviours | |
| Attitude | |

The Adult is that part of you that has gathered knowledge, experience and skills throughout your life. In the small child the Adult ego state is in a state of development and is sometimes called the Little Professor in that it acts on instinct, without the full experience and knowledge that you have as an adult, and often that instinct pays off. How we learn is the subject of psychological theory and I find Piaget's schematic process of development (as described in Gruber and Vonèche, 1977) useful in explaining how we learn to know and understand the world by building on past experiences, and the way in which we think qualitatively differently as a child compared with when we are an adult.

The Adult ego state learns how things work. It is the thinking part of the self. I think the perfect Adult ego state is presented by the character Mr Spock from the television and film series *Star Trek*. The character often considers his human colleagues as 'highly illogical' when they use emotional intelligence to help them get to the root of an intergalactic problem or when they express emotion such as love and hate. Please remember that Mr Spock is from another planet and as such does not represent a fully functioning human being, but I do call him to mind when I am struggling with an issue that needs level-headedness and rational, logical thought.

The Adult ego state is the bit of you that gets you organised. It makes plans, it formulates decisions and it weighs things up and remembers things. The Adult ego state relies on the direction of the parent and all those 'tape recorded' messages about what is right and what is wrong and it takes into account the feelings of the child. It has an executive function in deciding what to do.

### Recognising the Adult ego state

Like the Parent ego state, the Adult ego state is recognisable by the words, the tone, the behaviour and attitude used within an interaction. It asks questions like 'how?', 'when?', 'where?', 'who?' and 'why?' It uses phases such as 'that is interesting', 'mmm, I think that's a possibility' and 'maybe we could try that out'. The Adult ego state is calm, reflective and thoughtful and its attitude is one of being prepared to examine the facts, of level-headedness and rationality. The behaviour of the Adult ego state includes thoughtful looks, thinking behaviour, rubbing the face, scratching the head, gesturing possibilities with hand movements, itemising things and writing things down.

The Adult ego state can influence our Parent ego state by evaluating new information and instigating change through that reflective process. It can help to keep the emotions of the Child ego state in check but it is important to remember that the Adult ego state is a reflection of everything that has happened to us, so change is not always as easy as it sounds.

You will be familiar with sayings such as 'mind over matter' and you may believe that, if thought determines our behaviour, changing how people think will change their behaviour. However, if you have ever tried to change people's behaviour by using factual information and thoughts alone, you are likely to have been only partially successful. Let's examine that a little further.

**REFLECTION** 4.2

> How would you set about helping someone to give up smoking? You might also consider looking at other examples of risk-taking behaviour.

Changing someone's perception and behaviour isn't as easy as it sounds. You could try to give them new information that their Adult ego state could process, but it is more than likely that you will hit all sorts of obstacles that arise from the person's willingness to think things through.

Everyone knows that smoking poses an enormous health risk to the individual and those around them. To me the facts are quite clear, so why don't people stop smoking? Child ego state, feelings, ingrained patterns of behaviour and attitudes all need to be addressed. Just as you can rationalise the ways in which smoking is bad for them, someone else may rationalise that smoking didn't kill 'old Mr Smith' from down the road, who smoked 40 a day and lived till he was 103 years old, so it's not going to kill them and, besides that, they like it. The key to change is that people need to commit themselves to change and will need much more than factual information. We'll come back to this later.

## The Child ego state

Please don't assume that the word 'Child' means child-like. To be a fully functioning person we all need to be able to access our Child ego state. When we are born our Child ego state is all that we have. It is through the process of the 'parenting' of others that we develop other ego states. Berne (1961) argued that the Child ego state is, in many ways, the best bit of us. It is creative and joyful, it has fun and can be spontaneous, it is loving and uninhibited, it is curious, and in awe of the world. Not to have any of these aspects to our personality would leave the world bereft of all the things that have come out of these positive qualities. However, just as the Child has the potential for all these things, it is subject to its 'parenting' (I use the word 'parenting' to refer to the people who are responsible for parenting or care giving but may not be the child's parents in the biological sense).

The people who 'parent' the small child are all-powerful to that child and if their parenting skills, which are located and recorded in their Parent ego state, are not appropriate or fall short in some way, as a consequence of external or even internal events, the child still has to survive. To do so, the child adapts his/her behaviour. Adapted behaviour can be seen in all of us. Children are able to work out how to get what they want; their behaviour may please or displease their parents, but if the child wants attention it figures out the easiest and quickest way to get it. That way may involve kicking and screaming or doing something naughty like biting their baby sister, or it may be smiling nicely and looking up through ultra long lashes and being adorable. Either way attention is the result. That attention may not be delivered as we would like it to be, it may involve negative and harmful consequences, but attention is attention to the needy child. Our Child ego state adapts and learns how to manipulate situations, learns how to smile when unhappy, learns how to be cute, how to charm people and how to maintain the status quo. Not to adapt could result in tragedy for the personality as a whole, if not for the person, as it needs to be recognised that adaptive behaviour, while necessary to survive, can be very destructive and can result in devastating consequences.

The Child ego state holds all the feelings of childhood and carries them into adulthood where they continue to affect how we feel about ourselves and how we relate to others.

**WRITING ACTIVITY** 4.3

Repeat the same process as in *Writing activity 4.1* and see if you can identify the Child ego state characteristics.

| Characteristics | Natural/Free Child | Adapted Child |
|---|---|---|
| Words used | | |
| Tone of voice | | |
| Behaviours | | |
| Attitude | | |

### Child ego state words

The Child ego state often uses baby talk to express itself. It uses words like: 'help me', 'I can't do this on my own', 'this is my best day', 'my worst day', 'I can', 'I can't', 'I won't', 'I want', 'no', 'please', 'thank you', 'yippee', 'hooray', 'brilliant', 'yes', 'now', 'never'. Fitting them into what is free and what is adapted is a little tricky, but tone of voice is usually the giveaway. Tone of voice can often be in the extreme: screaming, shouting, excited, joyful, high-pitched or quiet, whining and pathetic.

### Child ego state behaviours

Child ego state behaviours reflect the emotions and feelings being experienced at the time. Folded arms, looking sad, giggling, not being able to give or maintain eye contact and hiding the face. Temper tantrums which involve thrashing arms and legs on the floor, etc. are common expressions of a Child ego state. Learning how to control extreme emotions is difficult but most of us manage it, although I do know a few adults who would love to kick and scream every now and then. The Child ego state knows how to hit your 'buttons' as they are able, through their Little Professor, to suss you out and to get you to react.

### Child ego state attitudes

Attitudes differ according to whether we are operating from our Free or Natural Child or from our Adapted Child. Child ego states can be free of inhibition, spirited, happy-go-lucky, volatile, manipulative, sly, cunning, compliant or defiant, all rolled up into one.

According to TA, 'good parenting' is the key to healthy Child ego states (Whitton, 1993) but healthy does not mean free or natural all of the time. We have to learn to self-regulate our behaviour and take our cues from others in order to fit in with our social group. Sometimes 'good parenting' is not possible because of our own parents' Parent ego state.

It may be damaged or incomplete. It is, after all, a product of its own experiences and maybe they did not have their emotional needs met when they were small. Being in our Parent ego state is comfortable as all those pre-recorded messages need little thinking about and little effort to sustain, but we can change those recorded ways of being through reflection and analysis of self and the relationships we have with others.

That was quite a tricky concept to explain and I did labour some of the points but it is important when using this framework to understand yourself and others, and not to attribute blame, as it takes two people to make a relationship. That brings me on nicely to transactions and communications between people.

# TRANSACTIONS BETWEEN PEOPLE

Alongside Structural Analysis of the personality, Eric Berne (1961) identified the process for analysing conversations between two or more people as the 'analysis of the transactional framework'. A transaction is said to be the means by which we receive and transmit 'strokes'. A stroke is defined as a 'unit of recognition' and strokes are essential to functional living. The achievement of strokes motivates our behaviour. According to this theory we all seek recognition from others. Recognition from others validates who we are. Transmitting a stroke to another person can be something as simple as saying 'good morning', and our reward is that they will say 'good morning' back, so validating that we are worthy of being recognised and responded to. When we give strokes we expect to be paid back.

## Complementary transactions

A transaction is transmitted and received via an ego state, and transactions are said to be either complementary, crossed or have at their core an ulterior motive. I've used one diagram (*Figure 4.1*) to show three examples of complementary transactions between the different ego states.

The Parent to Parent ego states are passing the time of day, sharing normal polite conversation. The Adult ego state is seeking information from another and receives the same. The Child issues an invitation to play which is accepted.

We are expected to pay back strokes by interacting with the person who gave us the stroke initially. A stroke may be a nod of the head or a series of strokes during a long discussion about global warming, but communication needs to be responded to in order for it to continue. If it is not responded to, the person who initiated the interaction often feels aggrieved. For example, if I say 'good morning' to a colleague and they don't respond I feel a bit put out. The Child ego state in my head says 'I must have done something' or 'she doesn't really like me' and I am left feeling embarrassed and sad. Later, I find myself sitting at the same table and I say, 'I said "hello" this morning and you totally ignored me. Have I offended you?' She responds immediately, 'Oh gosh no.

I am so sorry, my head was elsewhere this morning. I forgot my diary. I didn't see you. Anyway, how are you doing? You look absolutely great.' Not only do I get an apology and an explanation, but I also get an extra stroke in the form of a compliment. The communication between us can continue as she has paid back the stroke.

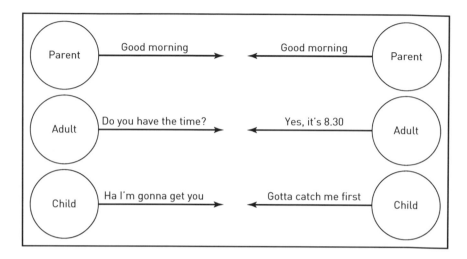

**Figure 4.1** *Complementary transactions between the different ego states.*

What if I hadn't caught up with her at lunch time but met someone else who had also been ignored by that person that morning? You can imagine the conversation. We talk about her ignoring us and decide she must be troubled by something and we agree to make a deliberate attempt to go find her and offer her our support, or we condemn her for being rude and ignorant and decide to ignore her in future (sounds like a Child ego state in play here). If a transaction is complementary it can continue. *Figure 4.2* gives other examples:

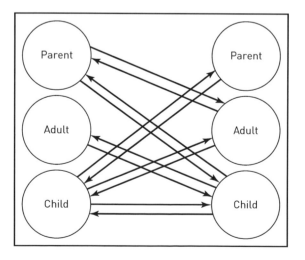
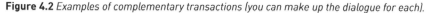

**Figure 4.2** *Examples of complementary transactions (you can make up the dialogue for each).*

## Crossed transactions

To be a complementary transaction one ego state must communicate with another and the response must come from the ego state the transaction was aimed at. This can go very wrong and, when it does, it is called a crossed transaction – see the examples in *Figure 4.3*.

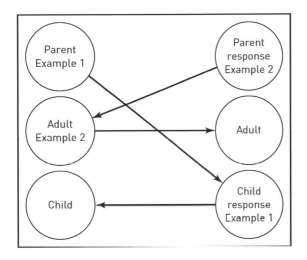

**Figure 4.3** *Crossed transactions.*

In *Figure 4.3* we can see a Parent ego state (Example 1) communicating with another person's Child ego state, shown via the diagrammatic line. It may be useful to note that the Parent ego state is likely to be a parent and the Child ego state is likely to be an actual child in this transaction. The Child ego state, rather than responding in a complementary way at the same level, chooses to respond by aiming its transaction to the other person's Child ego state in an adapted manner (Response 1).

Adding the following dialogue to the diagrammatic lines may help you to make sense of this crossed transaction.

**Parent 1:** When you have finished there you can come and have your tea.

**Child 1:** I don't want your stinky tea. I hate you and I hate tea, leave me alone.

The second example is that of an Adult ego state seeking information from another Adult ego state, but surprisingly the other person's Parent ego state responds. I've provided some dialogue as before but you may wish to add your own.

**Adult 2:** Do you know where the digital timer is?

**Parent 2:** Why do you expect me to know where everything is? You had it last.

Again, the response was not what was expected.

Crossed transactions often result in leaving people upset and the communication that was initiated ends as the invitation to come for tea or the request for information about the digital timer is left aside.

Berne (1972) calculated there were mathematically 72 types of crossed interactions and nine types of complementary interactions. I haven't been able to work them all out but, given his expertise, I believe it is so.

## Ulterior or covert transactions

The final type of transaction that Berne proposed is described as an ulterior or covert transaction. Here there is a social message in what is being said but there is a hidden message too (see *Figure 4.4*).

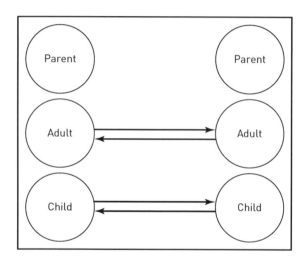

**Figure 4.4** *An ulterior or covert transaction.*

In this transaction the top line transaction represents the social level of the message sent Adult to Adult: 'Come up to the gallery and see my etchings …'. The response on a social level is Adult to Adult: 'Oh yes, that would be lovely'.

You can see in this transaction that there is another level of communication – Child to Child – referred to by Berne (1972) as the 'psychological' or 'covert level'. This sort of transaction has a psychological hook. In this example, that hook had a sexual connotation that has been recognised and accepted by the responder. However, the initiator took a risk as the responder could have responded from Critical Parent to Child with a comment such as: 'I don't particularly like etchings as I find them immature and brash.' The transaction would then be a crossed one and the communication ended.

# LIFE SCRIPTS

Another theory of TA is that of life scripts. It is suggested that, as small children, we write our own life script and then live according to its principles. A life script can be explored through the process of story-telling. Whitton (1993) provides an exercise to help explore life scripts. The following exercise is adapted from his text, *What is Transactional Analysis? A personal and practical guide.*

---

**REFLECTION AND WRITING ACTIVITY**

Think about your life as a small child and try to piece together a short story that describes your experience of the world and who you are. What happened when you were born? What did your parents say? Who gave you your name? Where do you fit in the family?

Write down a story that reflects your life. 500 words will do.

Reflecting on that story:

1. Are you the main character or do you have a cameo part?
2. Are you the hero or a drudge?
3. Is your story similar to other stories that you were fond of as a child?

---

The analysis of all this is up to you, but I hope it gives you an opportunity to think about who you are and how your childhood has influenced you as an adult. Perhaps it even helps to explain why you have chosen to be in the helping profession.

According to Whitton (1993), writing your life script took place before you were five years old. Life scripts influence how we receive and transmit messages to ourselves and to others. Our life script determines our decisions about what messages to accept and what to ignore. Life scripts, according to Whitton, are "essential for the child to survive". We hear stories of children who have been seriously abused or neglected but somehow they have raised themselves above all that negativity and become successful adults. According to this theory, these children wrote fantasy life scripts in their heads and used them to protect themselves from what went on around them. In this way they could refuse to receive negative messages and refuse to allow them to damage their personality, even though they may have been damaged physically. Positive messages would have been swept up, stored and cherished.

## I'm OK, You're OK

Very early in the writing of our life scripts we are said to make a decision about whether or not we are OK. The saying 'I'm OK, You're OK' may be familiar to you, and it originates from the title of a book written by Thomas Harris in 1969. Harris was an eminent psychiatrist and psychoanalyst and, as a TA practitioner, his work detailed how we respond to ourselves and to the world. Harris constructed the 'OK Corral' (see *Figure 4.5*) as a way of explaining people's Life Positions and concluded that, once we have made our life position decision, all our transactions are made in such a way as to maintain the same position.

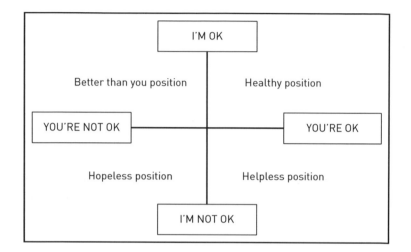

**Figure 4.5** *The OK Corral (Harris, 1969 and 1985).*

Where do you sit within the OK Corral? Each of us has a preferred way of being, and our transactions with the self and with others project this way of being. See if you can work out the following:

1.  Which position do the words 'Do as I say' come from?
2.  Which position do the words 'It's not fair' come from?
3.  Which position do the words 'That was fun, let's do it again' come from?
4.  Which position do the words 'Nobody can help me' come from?

I have no doubt you were able to work those positions out accurately as each ego state is clearly recognisable within the OK Corral, but I've included the answers at the end of the chapter for you to check.

That we make decisions about our life script and our life position at such an early stage is quite remarkable. According to TA theory we do review those decisions during adolescence but most of us stay the same and live our lives according to our script, taking selected strokes and messages as a reinforcement of our life position. On an intrapersonal level we call on those messages to help maintain the *status quo* even though they are not always healthy messages.

We are not always accurate in our understanding of life and we don't like change. Change brings with it anxiety and uncertainty and many people stay where they are, despite terrible consequences, as it is what they know. The Adult ego state within us is often contaminated by the other two ego states and rationalises situations in a flawed way, so maintaining life as it knows it to be.

Analysing transactions, life scripts and positions is fascinating and Eric Berne's explanation of the personality is easily understood. Once you learn how to identify which ego state you are operating from, you can understand why you behave and feel as you do. You could even choose to change your transaction by switching to another ego state. For example, you could move out of Critical Parent and stop criticising the children and join in their fun via your Child ego state. Knowing what ego state another person is in can help you to respond more effectively. You may even be able to intervene in such a way as to help the person understand which ego state they are operating from.

This chapter has introduced you to some of the principles of Transactional Analysis. TA provides a common language that you can share with others including family, friends, work colleagues and people that you seek to help. It is an effective communication tool as well as a psychotherapeutic technique and there are lots of texts available to read and courses to attend.

---

**READING ACTIVITY** 4.1

You need to read other people's accounts of Transactional Analysis, and TA practitioners are generally very generous in sharing their material. All of the books in the References are still in print and there are several websites that are worth having a look at such as, for example, www.itaa-net.org and www.ta-tutor.com

---

### Answers to Life Position questions

1. Which position do the words 'Do as I say' come from? Critical Parent in an I'm OK, You're not OK position.

2. Which position do the words 'It's not fair' come from? Adapted Child in a You're OK, I'm not OK position.

3. Which position do the words 'That was fun, let's do it again' come from? Free Child in an I'm OK, You're OK position.

4. Which position do the words 'Nobody can help me' come from? Adapted Child in an I'm not OK, You're not OK position.

> **CHAPTER SUMMARY**
>
> **Three key points to take away from Chapter 4:**
>
> - Transactional Analysis is an understandable theory that can be used by anyone as a method for understanding human communication and relationships.
> - TA proposes that our personality is made up of the Parent, Adult and Child ego states which each have different qualities and different patterns of behaviour and to be a fully functioning person, we need to have access to all of our ego states.
> - This simple model of personality can provide us with a powerful tool to analyse and gain insight into our and others' behaviour.

# FURTHER READING

www.ericberne.com/

Lapworth, P. and Sills, C. (2011) *An Introduction to Transactional Analysis: Helping people change.* London: Sage.

Whitton, E. (1993) *What is Transactional Analysis? A Personal and Practical Guide.* Essex, England: Gale Centre Publications.

# REFERENCES

Berne, E. (1957) *A Layman's Guide to Psychiatry and Psychoanalysis.* New York: Random House.

Berne, E. (1961) *Transactional Analysis in Psychotherapy.* New York: Grove Press.

Berne, E. (1968) *Games People Play. The psychology of relationships.* New York: Penguin Books.

Berne, E. (1972) *What Do You Say After You Say Hello?* New York: Corgi Press.

Berne, E. (1973) *Sex in Human Loving.* New York: Penguin Books.

Berne, E. (1977) *Intuition and Ego States. The origins of Transactional Analysis. A series of papers.* San Francisco: TA Press.

Gruber, H.E. and Vonèche, J.J. (eds) (1977) *The Essential Piaget.* New York: Basic Books.

Harris, T. (1969) *I'm OK, You're OK.* London: Pan Books.

Harris, T. (1985) *Staying OK.* London: Pan Books.

Klein, M. (1980) *Lives People Live. A Textbook of Transactional Analysis.* Chichester: Wiley Press.

Whitton, E. (1993) *What is Transactional Analysis? A personal and practical guide.* Essex, England: Gale Centre Publications.

# 05

# LISTENING TO PEOPLE

- Communication through listening

- The use of empathy

- Acceptance and non-judgemental warmth

- Being genuine

- Self-disclosure

- Active listening skills

- Confidentiality

- Knowing our limitations

## COMMUNICATION THROUGH LISTENING

We all know people who are confident and talkative. They will often dominate the conversation but we don't necessarily mind because they are amusing and engaging and it is great to have them at a social gathering because they have the ability to hold their audience and keep everyone entertained. We could say that they have good interpersonal skills, that they communicate well, but this would only be true if they could listen as well as they talked.

A fundamental part of effective communication is listening and the ability to show another person that they have been heard and understood. "Listening is more than the mere reception of sound. Listening is the basis for human interaction. It is deliberate, active behaviour" (Smith, 1986, p. 246). If you think about the people that you are most likely to go to when you feel you need to talk something through, you might well avoid the great raconteurs and go instead to someone who you know won't turn the conversation around to themselves but who will take an active interest in what you are saying. Rogers (1980, p. 12) describes the feeling of being truly listened to, saying: "These persons have heard me without judging me, diagnosing me, appraising me, evaluating me. They have just listened and clarified and responded to me at all levels at which I was communicating."

**REFLECTION** 5.1

Over the next few days spend some time observing those around you, both in your professional and personal life and focus on the way that people listen to you and others. How can you tell that you have been really heard? What does it feel like?

The kind of listening that we need to do will depend on our role and the kind of health or social care setting we work in. If we are assessing someone's needs or providing advice or information, we will need to listen specifically for factual information that will help us to provide the right kind of support. We might need to focus more on what a person means by what they are saying, so there will be a more interpretive quality to our listening. We might need to be listening at length to complex stories and information and helping the speaker to make sense of what they are saying or to help someone else understand what they are saying. Whatever kind of listening we are doing, it is an active and complex process and has the potential of supporting, respecting and often empowering the speaker.

Sometimes it is enough to listen sensitively, but at times when the people we are supporting are in distress, we need to listen in a way that shows we are willing to get to know them and 'walk alongside' them as they struggle to make sense of their experiences. This kind of listening has the potential to be therapeutic, it will benefit the speaker and contribute to their sense of emotional wellbeing. In many health and social care settings the people that we are supporting are likely to be vulnerable in some or many ways, so the way that we interact with them is vitally important and can make a significant difference to the way that they experience life and the situations they find themselves in.

**REFLECTION**

Think about your work setting: In what ways are the service users vulnerable?

You may have come up with some of the following:
- Elderly
- Living with illness
- Living with a disability: physical, learning or both
- A child, especially looked-after children
- Lonely or isolated
- Living with a mental illness
- Going through a difficult transition like bereavement, divorce or separation, losing their home, leaving home

- Homeless
- Asylum seeker or refugee.

It is not possible to write in detail in this book about the different kinds of listening we would need to do with so many different groups of people with so many different needs. There are specialist books which are listed at the end of this chapter which look at communicating with particular groups and give detailed advice. This chapter will focus on general active listening skills that underpin effective communication with all people regardless of their age or circumstances.

**ACTIVITY**

Find someone to do this activity with. Think of an experience you have had recently that was annoying or frustrating or upsetting. Tell your partner about the experience but while you talk they must make sure that they give you no indicators, whether verbal or non-verbal. They should avoid eye contact with you and make no response to what you are saying. Swap roles and ask them to tell you about something while you give them no indication that you are listening. Discuss the experience and the way that you each felt as you were talking.

Although this was an artificial exercise, it is quite probable that you felt some or all of the following:
- Invisible
- Unimportant
- Worthless
- Stupid
- Disrespected
- Ignored
- Upset
- Confused
- Angry

We have all experienced times in our life when things are going badly and it seems as if we will be overwhelmed with worries and we need someone who will listen. There are also times when we are happy, excited or proud and we want to share what has happened with someone. If we turn to someone who hasn't got the time to listen or who immediately starts to talk about their own worries or achievements it can impact negatively on our mood and our feelings about ourselves. In order to show that we are really listening rather than merely hearing, we need to be able to show that we have empathy for the speaker, that we accept them as they are without judging them, and we need to be genuine and honest. These three qualities are the foundations of the person-centred approach which was developed from the work of the psychologist Dr Carl Rogers (1902–1987).

Rogers developed Person-Centred Therapy which is an approach to counselling and psychotherapy but he came to believe that his ideas could be transferred to other areas where people were in relationships, like teaching, management, childcare and health and social care. In most settings where relationships are central to successful care, people use the work of Carl Rogers as the guiding principles in their approach. Working in this way relies not on specific techniques but on the personal qualities of the worker or helper and their ability to build positive relationships with others. This is why self-awareness and personal insight are so important, as we need to be able to separate our own feelings and experiences from those of the person we are helping so that we can listen to them as fully as possible.

## THE USE OF EMPATHY

Rogers described empathy as the ability to "sense the client's private world as if it were your own" (1957, p. 99). We show empathy or empathic understanding when we are able to spend some time in someone's shoes (metaphorically, of course) and show that we can see their world and understand their experiences as they have experienced them. When we are empathic we show our willingness to understand the uniqueness of someone else's experiences, thoughts and feelings. To be empathic we need to feel another's emotions without being overwhelmed by them. To extend the metaphor of being in someone else's shoes, we need to have one foot in the other person's shoe so that we feel and experience with them, whilst keeping the other foot firmly grounded in our own shoe.

Empathy should not be confused with sympathy or with telling someone you know how they feel. I'm sure there have been times when you have spoken to someone about your feelings of fear or anger or sadness and they respond with "I know what you mean, when that happened to me I ......" and they go on to talk about their experience rather than asking you more about your own. Sometimes you might need to talk about how confused you are about a situation and the person you are talking to says "Don't worry about it" or "Why don't you just ...." or "You ought to ..."These kind of responses, although well intentioned, simply make us feel that we haven't been heard and that our feelings are not important. It's very important to show that you accept and understand someone's feelings and thoughts before you jump in with your own thoughts, ideas or advice.

I remember a time when I was very low and found that I couldn't cope with a difficult situation in my life. I knew that I had to make important changes but felt completely stuck. My family and friends who I know cared deeply about me, offered lots of good advice and tried to comfort me by saying that everything would be OK but I just felt more and more miserable and less able to make changes. It was only when someone I didn't know very well allowed me to express how sad and angry and afraid of the future I was that I was able to feel less stuck. She simply listened to me and helped me to explore what had happened and the feelings I had. She showed me empathy and when I felt that I had really been understood, I was able to start to make changes.

**REFLECTION** **5.2**

Think of the following scenario: The father of a child aged fifteen who has profound and multiple learning difficulties is struggling to care for him at home. He is a single parent whose wife left when their child was five and who no longer sees them. He works part-time and enjoys his job. He has help provided by social services but this is only on the days that he is at work. He is considering moving his son to a residential setting. To all the services and professionals that he comes into contact with he appears to be a positive and competent parent, coping well and uncomplaining. If possible, discuss with a partner and make a list of the feelings that he is likely to be experiencing at this time of transition.

## Discussion

He is likely to be *exhausted* much of the time because of the physical demands of his now adolescent son. He might feel *confused* about his decision, unsure about whether it is the right thing to do. The confusion is possibly tinged with *guilt* as he feels that he is giving up on his son, that he should be the one to care for him. He might also feel guilty that he enjoys his job; that it gives him brief respite from the physical and emotional demands of caring for his son. If we look deeper into his experiences as a parent he might feel a deep *sadness* that his son's life is so much more difficult than other children of his age, that he will never be independent. He might feel *grief* at the loss of the life he thought that he and his son would have if he hadn't been born with such difficulties. There might also be a sense of *fear* that he might become too old to care for his son and that he might die before his son. There is likely to be *anger* and *resentment* at his ex-wife who left him and their son. He might feel a lot of *pride*, always having strived to show people that he is coping and can provide for his son's needs.

This example should give you an idea of the complexity of people's lives and of the importance of empathy when we are working with people who are experiencing difficulties like this. This man is having to make a really difficult decision that will have a huge impact on him and the life of his son. In order to support him, the professionals working with him need to be aware of the multitude of feelings he might be having and strive to understand his unique situation as he makes his decision.

Showing empathic understanding of people's lives and experiences is an essential part of listening and effective communication and, as stated before, much depends on the personal qualities of the listener but there are particular skills that can be learnt and used to communicate empathy. Later in this chapter you will find out about how to listen to people in an empathic way through the use of active listening skills.

# ACCEPTANCE AND NON-JUDGEMENTAL WARMTH

Rogers (1957) called this non-judgemental and accepting attitude 'unconditional positive regard'. It is an attitude which communicates to another person that you accept them as they are without conditions. Nelson Jones (2011, p. 104) suggests alternative terms such as "non-possessive warmth, caring, prizing, acceptance and respect". It is logical that if we are to show empathy to someone, we also need to show them that we accept them as they are with warmth and without judgement. We need to communicate that we are willing to respect and accept someone's ideas, thoughts and feelings even when we don't understand or agree with them.

**REFLECTION** 5.3

Think about a time when you felt that someone was judging you. It might be because you made a decision that they didn't agree with or you had an opinion that was different to theirs. How did they show their judgement of you? How did it affect you and your feelings? How did you respond?

Many of us are our own harshest critics and we judge ourselves and anticipate criticism from others. However, if we feel that we are being judged by others, particularly a professional to whom we come for support, we are likely to experience a combination of these feelings: embarrassed, ashamed, angry, defensive, upset, worthless, anxious, misunderstood, disrespected, unsure, confused. When we experience negative feelings like these we are unlikely to feel understood or supported in any way. Instead, depending on our personality, if we feel embarrassed or upset we are likely to withdraw and avoid further discussion, we might even avoid that person altogether, especially if they are a professional that we don't have to come into contact with. Alternatively, we might feel defensive and annoyed; we will want to argue our position and reject any offers of support or advice. If we are confused and unsure we are far less likely to feel any confidence in our opinions – we feel stuck and unable to make changes or take decisions that will benefit us. Being judged can only affect our self-esteem negatively.

Having emphasised the importance of not judging people it is necessary to acknowledge how difficult it is to achieve. To be completely non-judgemental is an ideal that I would argue is impossible to reach. As humans we cannot help but have opinions about certain things. As we saw in *Chapter 2*, we all have different values and beliefs depending on our culture and environment and we cannot help but have views that are at odds with those of others and end up judging them based on our own values. In both our personal and professional lives, in order to be more accepting we need to be curious about how people's values and beliefs were formed and how they impact on their thoughts and behaviour. The following scenario illustrates how we might show this:

Imagine you see a mother shout angrily at her small child who accidentally drops something. Depending on your own values, you might find it difficult not to feel angry, sad, disapproving, shocked or concerned. Of course it would be hard not to judge this behaviour negatively but if you took time to think about what that mother's experience is, we might find that we are judgemental about her actions but less so about her as an individual. If that were to happen in a Children's Centre and you were a worker there, you might feel the urge to criticise the mother for shouting at her child but this is unlikely to help her. She will immediately feel judged and will either be angry or upset. She might avoid you, perhaps refusing to attend the Centre again. If you respond to her in a non-judgemental and empathic way by acknowledging the feelings of anger and stress which led to her actions she is more likely to feel accepted and might be able to reflect on her actions if she feels safe and supported.

**REFLECTION** 5.4 &#9000;

Think about situations in your work setting where you feel that people, especially service users, are judged negatively. How do you think they respond to this? How might the practitioners behave or speak in a less judgemental, more accepting way? The section on active listening skills will help you to do this.

## BEING GENUINE

Being empathic and accepting are vitally important but they are very difficult to show unless we are also genuine, honest and fully ourselves when we are listening to people who need support. Rogers (1957) called this genuineness 'congruence' and it describes a way of being in which we are our authentic selves, without pretence or façade. If we are real and genuine with others then they are far more able to be real and genuine with us. Think about situations when you are with someone who is in authority – you might feel intimidated and anxious, concerned about the impression that you are making. This is often the case when we go to see a doctor or manager or head teacher; if they are the kind of person who feels they need to assert their authority or their knowledge and expertise, it can be difficult to talk openly and honestly about our concerns. If on the other hand they make us feel at ease by dropping the façade of authority, showing a genuine interest in us, responding to what we say with empathy and acceptance, we are more likely to feel supported.

Being genuine doesn't mean that we should blurt out everything we are thinking or feeling. Rather, it means we should share the parts of ourselves and our thoughts that are relevant and helpful to the other person and beneficial to the relationship. If someone is telling us about a situation that makes us angry, we could tell them "I can feel a real tension in my body as you tell me that, it must have been such a difficult situation for you". This genuineness allows the speaker to feel that you are really with them and it will help them to open up further. However we shouldn't tell people how we feel if it is not going to benefit them. It might be honest to tell someone that they are boring or irritating but it is not helpful, nor will it make them feel supported. Our feelings of boredom or irritation are our own responsibility and we need to reflect on why we might feel that way.

As with acceptance, it is not possible to be genuine at all times; we cannot be perfectly real and open all the time. Of course we need to protect ourselves and others by keeping our feelings and thoughts to ourselves if they are likely to damage the relationship but we can strive to be as fully present in the moment as possible. We might be feeling stressed and angry and irritated and want to speak in an abrupt and dismissive way to someone but this would inevitably damage the relationship. It is better to say something like: "I'm not sure that I'm able to listen to you properly at the moment as my head feels full of all sorts of other stuff and I don't think I'd be very helpful to you. I will come back as soon as I can." This is genuine without being insensitive and it shows that you are taking responsibility for your own feelings.

There will be times when we find it impossible to be non-judgemental and genuine at the same time, especially when someone behaves in a cruel or bullying way, has prejudiced and bigoted views or is critical and judgemental of others. We need to be able to separate the views and behaviour from the person and respond appropriately. It is possible to be both genuine and accepting at the same time. We might say something like: "I found it really uncomfortable when you were shouting at Mrs Smith and I was wondering what was going on for you at that point. I thought maybe it was difficult for you to have to spend time with someone you don't like?" A response like this encourages the speaker to explore their feelings rather than attempt to defend or justify their actions and it also allows the listener to be honest about their discomfort.

## SELF-DISCLOSURE

If we are effective in establishing positive, helping relationships with service users, it will sometimes be appropriate to offer some personal information about ourselves. This is called self-disclosure and it takes place when a helper is willing to share relevant and significant personal information with a service user. When shared appropriately this can be used to:

- encourage the service user to say what they want to;
- show them that they are not alone in their feelings and/or experiences;
- demonstrate your own humanity.

You should be aware that there are dangers here and I feel that it is better not to use self-disclosure at all than to over-use it. Where there is an over-sharing of personal information it can:

- take the emphasis away from the service user;
- create an impression of what I call 'been there, done that, got the T-shirt', which can undervalue the experiences of the service user.

Each one of us needs to decide what, if anything, we are willing to share from our personal lives. This can then be used in a controlled way to benefit the service user. For example, you might work with those who are struggling to come to terms with the death of someone that they loved. If you have experienced this yourself, individuals might find it helpful for you to tell them a little of your feelings and coping strategies following the death of someone close to you. This seems to help in a number of ways:

- They can see that it is possible to endure the pain of bereavement
- It can normalise their own response to death
- It can help them to feel that their pain is understood
- It may help them project to a time when they too will be able to live life again.

In your personal relationships, you will probably not even think about the amount of information that you disclose about yourself because family relationships, friendships and the relationships we have with colleagues are different from those that we have with those in our care. Self-disclosure is often unnecessary as you are interested in their lives and experiences rather than your own; however, if we are to be genuine and real, a certain amount of self-disclosure is natural but it should be limited and it should be of use to the person you are listening to.

## ACTIVE LISTENING SKILLS

It is agreed by most professionals working in health and social care that a person-centred approach is an essential component of support. Indeed, the Core Competencies for Healthcare Support Workers and Adult Social Care Workers include "Person-centred care and support" (Skills for Care, 2013). Being empathic, accepting and genuine are therefore essential qualities for health and social care workers but how do we actually communicate these qualities to the people that we are supporting? The quality of the relationship is the most important part of effective listening and communication and this cannot be taught or learnt but there are certain skills which help to foster emotional wellbeing and promote a positive and therapeutic relationship.

### Body language

A very important part of our body language is eye contact which has been covered in *Chapter 3*. This section will look at other aspects of our non-verbal communication.

### Observing the body language of the speaker

Body language is very important and can tell us a lot about what is going on for the person we are listening to. In order to show that we are listening and are able to empathise when someone is talking to us, we need to notice what their body language is telling us as well as their words. Open body language communicates a willingness to talk and listen. It is relaxed with good eye contact with the body positioned towards you. The arms and legs are usually uncrossed. Closed body language might communicate a lack of willingness to talk or listen. Eye contact will be poor, with the person looking away and possibly positioning their body away from you. They might have their arms crossed, defending their body or be completely hunched over, making themselves as small as possible. They might be fidgeting or completely withdrawn and still. Sometimes the body language will look open but it will be tense: eye contact is too intense, fists are clenched and the chest is pushed out in an attempt to appear more threatening. This suggests an aggressive or antagonistic attitude. *Chapter 6* will look at managing strong emotions such as anger.

It is especially important to notice when there is a mismatch between what someone is saying and what their body language suggests. If someone is telling you they are fine but their face is turned away from you and their fists are clenched it would suggest that they are upset or angry. If they are wringing their hands or fiddling with their clothing or hair or jewellery it might suggest that they are anxious. When the body language is at odds with the verbal message it is important to be tentative with our approach. We cannot make people talk to us – we must respect their right to stay silent but equally we should communicate our willingness to listen if they do want to talk. Saying something like "You seem to be a bit worried/upset, have I got that right? We could have a talk now if you'd like or later if you feel that you need to." This allows them to accept or decline the invitation or to have the space to decide if they are ready to talk.

### Awareness of our own body language

It is equally important for us to be aware of our own body language and think of what messages we are sending to the person we are talking to. Egan (2002, p. 69) suggests a useful acronym which helps us to think about our body language when we are in a helping role.

**S:** face the client *Squarely*

**O:** adopt an *Open* posture

**L:** remember that it is possible to *Lean* towards the other

**E:** maintain good *Eye* contact

**R:** try to be relatively *Relaxed* or natural in these behaviours.

This is a really useful way of keeping the importance of body language in mind but there may be times when you feel that you need to loosen these guidelines because you want the person you are helping to feel as relaxed as possible. You should try to maintain an open posture to show your availability and willingness to listen. If the person is sitting, it is important for you to be sitting too. If you are sitting or standing make sure that you leave enough personal space between you to avoid intimidating or making the person feel uncomfortable. If you are sitting, your chairs should be angled towards each other rather than squarely opposite as that could feel like an interrogation. Sometimes if the person seems a bit shy or withdrawn and finds it hard to make eye contact you could sit at a table alongside them and join in or suggest an activity that you could do together. This can make the atmosphere more relaxed and if the person feels unsure what to say or needs space to think, it can feel easier if you are side by side, engaged in another activity so the pressure is off. It is sometimes best with eye contact and body language to try to mirror the person you are talking to whilst encouraging openness. If they are leaning back in their chair in a relaxed way it would be strange for you to be sitting straight up with a stiff spine. If they find it difficult to make eye contact, you should try not to direct your gaze towards them too much of the time.

## Acknowledging and reflecting feelings

Feelings and emotions are words that are often used synonymously but it might be useful to distinguish between the two. Feltham and Dryden (1993) suggest that feelings are experienced and emotions are exhibited. This can make it difficult to recognise the feeling that a person is experiencing. They might be exhibiting an emotion of anger but actually experiencing intense sadness. Earlier in this chapter we discussed the importance of showing empathy and being able to understand someone's feelings and experiences. In order to do this it is important for people to feel that their feelings have been recognised and acknowledged, and that their thoughts and worries are valued, but this can be hard to do if the emotions they are showing are hiding their true feelings.

Think back to *Reflection 5.2*, about the father who has a child with profound and multiple learning disabilities. The father might be experiencing a combination or all of the feelings highlighted in the discussion, and he might express them in different ways. If he says that he is angry or guilty or sad it is important that those feelings are validated. Sometimes we can find it hard to listen to the intensity of someone's sadness, guilt, anger or frustration and our reaction in this example might be to say "Don't cry", "Calm down" or "Don't worry". Although our motivation might be to comfort him, we are in fact telling him not to show or even feel what he is feeling.

Being listened to and having the space to explore confused feelings with someone who isn't going to tell us to stop feeling angry or sad or afraid, can help us to process our feelings and feel better about ourselves. It is important, when talking to a person about what they are going through, that we listen for the feelings, even when they are not labelled specifically. It is often the case that someone doesn't know how they are feeling. They can't identify the bad feeling they have. It might be anger, fear or sadness but they might need someone who can recognise the feeling and help them to express and process it.

Sometimes people will tell you how they feel without any prompting. When this happens you need to reflect that feeling back to them. "I was furious with him for selling my stuff". You could simply repeat the word 'furious' which invites the speaker to say more or you could say "It must have made you really angry".

Sometimes you will not hear a feeling word and need to use your empathic understanding to try to gauge how someone is. The most obvious way of acknowledging feelings is to ask the person how they are actually feeling. You can simply say "How did you feel when that happened?" Sometimes they will tell you and you can go on to explore that by saying something like: "Tell me a bit more about that" or "How long has it felt like this for you?"

Often they will not tell you directly but you can tell that something isn't right. You might then say something like:

"I'm wondering if you're feeling angry about what happened this morning?"

"It sounds like you're feeling sad about what happened with your daughter"

"I'm guessing it would have been really upsetting when you had to pack up your house and move here".

When you offer a suggestion of how a person might be feeling you give them the opportunity to accept or reject those feelings. They might reply "No, I'm not sad, I'm more angry than sad" and so through the process of exploring those feelings you are enabling them to understand them more clearly. Rogers describes the way he checks his understanding with the client as "catching just the colour and texture and flavour of the personal meaning you are experiencing right now" (Rogers, 1986, p. 125).

As a final note on acknowledging feelings, it is very important to consider the culture of the people we work with. Emotions and expressions of emotions are subjective and dependent on the context of the speaker and listener and may reflect the socio-cultural norms of both. It is important to understand a culture if we are to understand the emotions that are expressed by people of that culture (Banerjee, 2005). If we have little understanding of a culture, it's fine to be curious about what might be going on for a person. You could say something like "I noticed that when John took your phone away you didn't seem at all annoyed, did you feel annoyed?"

## Paraphrasing

Paraphrasing is the skill of rephrasing the important parts of what you have heard someone say. It is a way of showing that you understand their point of view. We often feel the need to offer solutions or advice and sometimes this is just what people want but it is important that you show your understanding of their situation and acknowledge their feelings before jumping in with solutions or advice. It is usually true that people need to find the solutions that work best for them. In using this skill you will:

- Check your understanding of what they have said
- Communicate the core qualities of acceptance and empathic understanding
- Gain information about how they see themselves and their concerns
- Build a trusting relationship (Culley and Bond, 2004).

You need to be accurate when paraphrasing. Sometimes you might get it wrong so if you are not sure you can offer the paraphrase tentatively, using phrases like "It sounds like...." or "It seems that......" or "I'm wondering if I've got that right."

An example of paraphrasing would be:

*Service user:* I can't believe I have to wait another six weeks for an assessment. It feels like no one cares about me or my situation. I'm so tired and irritated all the time. I'm snapping at my kids and my colleagues at work and it's not their fault, it just pops out before I have a chance to stop myself.

*Helper:* It sounds like your frustration with having to wait is spilling out so as well as feeling angry, you feel guilty too.

If someone does go on to ask your advice, it can be tempting to offer it straight away, but having shown your understanding of their situation you could then just ask "What have you thought of already?" "What do you feel all the options are?" This enables them to explore the ideas they already have and to feel supported and listened to as they find their way.

## Summarising

Summaries are longer paraphrases and enable you to bring together in an organised way the important aspects of what a person has said (Culley and Bond, 2006). Quite often a person might want to talk about many things that are on their mind, especially when life feels overwhelming. They might talk in quite a chaotic way, jumping from one subject to another, digressing and changing their tone of voice. This can make it quite difficult to follow but it's often a reflection of the chaos in their lives. Summarising is useful when the conversation is coming to an end or when they've talked for quite a long time, as it can help you both to clarify what is going on. It can also serve to organise and prioritise what the problems and issues are. Here is an example of a summary that a family support worker uses after talking to a mother who is struggling to cope.

"So it sounds like your problems are overwhelming you. Your ex-husband isn't giving you any financial support and rarely has the children to stay. Your friends are caught up in their own problems and can't help. Your children are arguing all the time and on top of that your hours at work have been cut and money is even tighter. I'm wondering which of these feels like it's taking up the most space in your head at the moment?"

This summary allows the woman to hear the issues that she is facing and to feel that someone understands the pressure she is under. By simply summarising what she has said, she is given the opportunity to reflect on her situation without someone else offering their opinion.

Culley and Bond (2004) offer the following guidelines for paraphrasing and summarising:
- Be tentative and offer your perception of what the client has said
- Avoid telling, informing or defining the client
- Be respectful, do not judge, dismiss or use sarcasm
- Use your own words; repeating verbatim may seem like mimicry
- Listen to the depth of feeling expressed and match the level in your response
- Do not add to what the client says, evaluate it or offer interpretations
- Be congruent and don't pretend you understand
- Be brief and direct
- Keep your voice tone level. Paraphrasing in a shocked or disbelieving tone will communicate neither acceptance nor empathy.

## Questioning

There are many different kinds of questions which elicit many different responses, and it can be difficult to know what to ask and what impact the questioning might have on a person who might be confused and distressed. More often than not it is enough to just listen without questioning. It is surprising how much we can learn by simply using reflection and paraphrasing. However, if our role requires us to gather information or to help someone with something specific we will have to ask questions.

There are two main kinds of questions: open and closed.

**Open questions** – these are often questions which beginning with 'what', 'where', 'how', and 'who'. These are the most useful kinds of questions as they involve the person more and encourage exploration and thoughtfulness. Try to avoid 'why' questions as they put pressure on the person to justify their position.

**Closed questions** – these invite the person to answer 'yes' or 'no'; they are non-exploratory and tend to cut discussion short.

Look at these examples of open and closed questions and see how they might elicit very different responses.

| Open | Closed |
|------|--------|
| How are you feeling today? | Are you feeling better today? |
| What did you want to be when you were young? | Did you always want to be a nurse? |
| What was it like for you when he refused to do what you asked? | Were you annoyed when he refused to do what you asked? |
| What did you like about living abroad? | Did you like living abroad? |

In general it is better to use open questions but some people find it difficult to express themselves or are shy or reluctant to say much. At times like this it is advisable to use closed questions at the beginning because they are much less threatening and complex and they can enable you to at least get a sense of what is going on for the person you are speaking to. As they feel more comfortable it is likely that they will give fuller, more detailed answers.

## Listening to silence

Silence can be awkward and threatening and uncomfortable but we can learn a lot from what people do not say as well as from what they do say. It is important to allow silences when we are talking to people who need support. It is natural in normal conversation to try to fill silences but in therapeutic communication it is essential to allow space for the person to process their thoughts. You might have experienced times in your life when things are overwhelming and you don't even know how to feel let alone express your thoughts. It can be very comforting to know that someone is with you, supporting you but not demanding that you speak. When this happens it might well be enough for you to have a safe place to think, in the presence of someone who is trusted and undemanding. As listeners we can show that we are emotionally available to someone by our non-verbal communication, our open and relaxed body language, our attentiveness through eye contact. It might be that they never open up but that they still seek you out – it's important to trust that they are benefiting from your presence.

## Listening to people who are having suicidal thoughts

When someone is extremely distressed and starts to talk about ending their life it can be very difficult to manage without getting upset yourself or sometimes panicking and trying to find a way out of the situation. Sometimes despair can lead to suicidal thoughts. We might be working with people who are in very difficult circumstances, they are depressed and feel that life is too difficult. When people feel helpless or hopeless it may seem as if the only way to manage these feelings is to know that death is within their control. If you are with someone who expresses a wish to take their own life, either directly by saying "I want to kill myself" or indirectly by saying something like "I just don't feel I can go on any more", it is very important that you take it seriously. It should never be minimised or seen as a cry for help. Talking with someone about their suicidal thoughts doesn't make it more likely that they will do something to end their life. Instead you should stay with them and encourage them to talk and use active listening skills, showing them your willingness to understand what they are experiencing and feeling. You should discuss strategies for help like seeing their GP, phoning the Samaritans or in extreme circumstances, if they are talking about ending their life imminently, going to Accident and Emergency so that they can get appropriate support straight away. If someone discloses that they are having suicidal thoughts it is usually because they want help so it is important that you talk to a line manager or mentor or supervisor to discuss the most appropriate way of helping. If someone in your care is in a distressed state or clearly depressed you need to be aware of your limitations both professionally and personally, recognising that they need more specialised support and knowing who to refer on to.

**WRITING ACTIVITY** ( 5.1 )

Here is a short script of an interaction that might be quite typical in a care home setting. Read through it and write notes on the following:

1. What do you think are the feelings being experienced by both Jane and the care worker?

2. How do you think the care worker's responses impact on Jane and her feelings at this time?

3. Write out the script again using appropriate active listening skills.

CARE WORKER (putting down a cup of tea): Here you go Jane.

JANE: Thanks, have you got a minute? It'd be nice to have some company, it's all so strange here after my lovely little house.

CW: Does it have to be now? I'm run off my feet.

J (upset): Sorry, I didn't mean to be a bother. It's OK, you get on love. I'll be OK, I seem to be getting in everyone's way lately.

CW: I'll see if I can come back later.

CW (later on): Right Jane, I've got a minute or two, what was it you wanted?

J: I don't want to put you out.

CW: Well I'm here now. What was it you said earlier about it being strange here? Don't you like it?

**WRITING ACTIVITY** 5.1 CONT'D

J: Yes, I suppose I'm just a bit homesick.

CW: At your age? Don't be silly, you'll be fine.

J: Yes, maybe. I didn't really want to come into this home but my son and daughter didn't think they could go on helping out on a daily basis so they thought it would be for the best for me to come here.

CW: Well it can be hard caring for an elderly relative, I should know. It's probably for the best. You don't have to worry about bothering them and they aren't burdened with the responsibility. You'll settle in in no time. You've got a lovely room with a lot of your stuff in it. People like me at your beck and call – life of Riley!!!! But seriously, I know it can be hard at first – but chin up – look on the bright side.

J: Yes, I suppose so. Off you go dear, I've taken up enough of your time already.

CW: Bye then, see you later.

## Things to remember about active listening skills

| Active listening skill | Key points |
|---|---|
| Body language | Be aware of your own body language and the effect it has on the person you are listening to. |
| | Use open body language as this communicates your willingness to listen. |
| | Be aware of the body language of the person you are listening to, and in particular observe any mismatch between what they are saying and what their body language is conveying. |
| Acknowledging and reflecting feelings | Show that you have empathy for the person who is talking to you by acknowledging their feelings and reflecting back that understanding to them. Don't contradict or minimise the feeling when someone tells you how they feel, even if it feels uncomfortable. |
| Paraphrasing | Show your understanding of what has been said by offering a short summary of what you have heard. This enables the speaker to reflect on what they have said. |
| Summarising | When someone has been speaking for a while and has brought up a few points and concerns, summarise what they have said so that they know you have understood. Offering a summary also enables the speaker to focus on the most significant issue. |

*(continued)*

| Active listening skill | Key points |
|---|---|
| Questioning | Try not to ask too many questions; reflecting and paraphrasing usually helps the speaker to clarify what they have said. Open questions are more useful than closed questions because they encourage more exploration. |
| Listening to silence | Don't be afraid of silence; allowing silence and being present with your eye contact and body language gives the speaker time to reflect and process what they are saying. It shows an empathy for their situation without asking them to explain what they are thinking or feeling. |
| Listening to people who are having suicidal thoughts | Do not minimise what the person is saying; continue to use all the above active listening skills. Seek support from a line manager as soon as feels appropriate, making sure that the person doesn't leave your care. |

**WRITING ACTIVITY** 5.2

Spend a week keeping a journal of the different interactions that you have had with friends, family, work colleagues and particularly any service users that you come into contact with. Focus specifically on how well you have listened. Try to use some of the active listening skills that are suggested in this chapter and reflect on how they affected the interactions you had.

## CONFIDENTIALITY

Trust and confidentiality are two of the most important values in health and social care settings. Trust has to be at the foundation of any good relationship and is an important part of effective communication. If people feel that their privacy might be violated by a health and social care professional they are unlikely to want to use the services that they need. Our ability to show that we can be trusted and relied on is an important interpersonal skill. The Ethical Framework for Good Practice in Counselling and Psychotherapy (2007) stresses the importance of confidentiality. The Nursing and Midwifery Council Code of Conduct (2012) states that: "You must respect people's right to confidentiality." It is therefore extremely important that you reassure the people that you work with at the outset of your relationship with them, that what they tell you will be kept confidential.

However, alongside our duty to keep what a person is telling us confidential, is our duty to keep them and others safe from harm. As health and social care professionals we are duty bound to adhere to safeguarding policies and practices and so confidentiality is only possible if what people are telling us is within the law. All public agencies recognise that there some situations when a person's right to confidentiality is compromised. If we hear about a vulnerable person, adult or child, whose safety is being put at risk, who is being abused or neglected, we have an obligation to report it. Your work setting will have safeguarding policies and practices which you must become familiar with and follow if you hear of any vulnerable person who is not safe. Your supervisor, mentor or line manager must be told and then they will contact an appropriate agency such as the police, Children's Services or social workers responsible for protecting vulnerable people.

Moss (2012) provides helpful guidance on how to raise the issue of confidentiality with a person that you are beginning to work with. I have adapted it to fit with most situations in health and social care settings and acknowledge that you as an individual might not be able to offer confidentiality if you are in training or have to share what you do with someone else:

"Hello, before we get started I need to explain a few things to you about confidentiality. I hope that you realise that I (and the other people that work here) will work with you with the utmost respect and what you say to me/us will not be shared with anyone else/ outside this setting. But, there are some occasions with some people when they tell us something which we can't keep to ourselves. The sort of thing I mean is when we hear about children or vulnerable adults being abused or put at risk. If we hear about that sort of thing, we are legally bound to inform social workers or the police. I'm sure you appreciate the importance of that. We will always seek your consent before we speak to someone else about you and if we did feel that we needed to contact someone else, we would tell you what we were going to do. I hope that you have understood how important this is." (Moss, 2012, p. 73)

## CHAPTER SUMMARY

### Ten key points to take away from Chapter 5:

- A fundamental interpersonal skill is listening and the ability to show another person that they have been heard and understood. Good relationships are the bedrock of good communication.
- The experience of being listened to can be therapeutic and beneficial to our emotional wellbeing.
- It is particularly important that vulnerable people in our care are listened to and responded to in a supportive, caring and respectful way.
- Rogerian person-centred principles of empathy, acceptance and genuineness are at the foundations of effective listening and care.
- Empathy is the ability to experience another's feelings and experiences as if they were our own.

> **CHAPTER SUMMARY CONT'D**
>
> - Acceptance and non-judgemental warmth are essential for our sense of self-worth.
> - Genuineness and the ability to be fully ourselves whilst remaining professional are a key part of building trusting therapeutic relationships.
> - We show these person-centred qualities through the use of active listening skills which can be learnt and practised.
> - Confidentiality is an important part of trust but must be offered within professional safeguarding boundaries.
> - We must know when to refer on to a more specialised service when the people in our care need more support.

## USEFUL READING

Any book on counselling skills would be useful to you. For general skills the following books are useful:

Burnard, P. (1989) *Teaching Interpersonal Skills. A handbook of experiential learning for health professionals*. London: Chapman and Hall.

Culley, S. and Bond, T. (2004) *Integrative Counselling Skills in Action*. London: Sage Publications.

For information on listening and counselling skills in specific settings, the following books might be useful:

*For those working with children and young people:*

McLeod, A. (2008) *Listening to Children – A practitioner's guide*. London: Jessica Kingsley Publishers.

Geldard, K. and Geldard, D. (2010) *Counselling Adolescents: The proactive approach for young people*. London: Sage.

*For those working with people with Alzheimer's and dementia:*

Feil, N. and Klerk-Rubin, V. (2012) *The Validation Breakthrough: Simple techniques for communicating with people with Alzheimer's and other dementias* 3rd ed. Baltimore: Health Professions Press.

The Alzheimer's Society has very useful guidelines for communicating with people with dementia. You can find these at:

www.alzheimers.org.uk/site/scripts/documents_info.php?documentID=130

*For those working with people with a learning disability:*

Thurman, S. (2011) Communicating effectively with people with a learning disability. Exeter: Learning Matters Ltd and Kidderminster: BILD.

*Or specifically for people with autism:*

The National Autistic Society website (www.autism.org.uk) has a really useful section at: www.autism.org.uk/living-with-autism/communicating-and-interacting/communication-and-interaction.aspx

# REFERENCES

Banerjee, R. (2005). *Cultural Differences in the Experience and Expression of Emotion.* Social and Emotional Aspects of Learning: Guidance. DfES.

Culley, S. and Bond, T. (2004). *Integrative Counselling Skills in Action.* London: Sage Publications.

Egan, G. (2002) *The Skilled Helper* 7th ed. Pacific Grove: Brooks/Cole.

Feltham, C. and Dryden, W. (1993). *Dictionary of Counselling.* London: Whirr Publishers.

Moss, B. (2012) *Communication Skills in Health and Social Care.* London: Sage.

Nelson Jones, R. (2011) *The Theory and Practice of Counselling and Therapy* 5th ed. London: Sage.

Rogers, C. (1957) The Necessary and Sufficient Conditions for Therapeutic Change. *Journal of Consulting Psychology*, **21:** 95–103.

Rogers, C. (1980) *A Way of Being.* New York: Houghton Mifflin Company.

Rogers, C. (1986) Reflection of Feelings. *Person Centred Review*, **1(4):** 125–140.

Skills for Care (2013) Core Competencies for Healthcare Support Workers and Adult Social Care Workers. Leeds: Skills for Care and Skills for Health.

Smith, V. (1986) Listening. In Hargie, O (ed.) *A Handbook of Communication Skills.* London: Routledge.

# 06

# COMMUNICATION AND INTERPERSONAL SKILLS IN PRACTICE

**KEY THEMES:**

- Things that are important to people
- Blocks and barriers to effective communication
- Dealing with difficult people
- Working and communicating with others in organisations
- Communication through the written word
- Using telephone, email and mobile phones
- Using social media.

## THINGS THAT ARE IMPORTANT TO PEOPLE

As a student working or intending to work in a health or social care setting you will find it useful to spend some time reflecting upon what it is like to be at the receiving end of the care that you and your organisation offer. To begin the work of *Chapter 6*, I would like to ask you what you think are the most important things in your life.

**REFLECTION** 6.1

Think about all those things that are really important to you. They may be tangible things that you own, or they may be abstract ideas or considerations that you hold to be of value to yourself and others. You might wish to take your time over this reflective activity, sharing your thoughts and ideas with those people close to you and perhaps extending that to the people you study and work with.

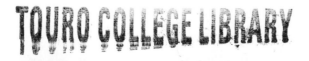

**REFLECTION** 6.1 CONT'D

Having reflected on those issues most dear to you, I would now like you to identify a list of twenty of the most important things to you in the world but, before you do that, I am going to impose some limits on what can be held in your list:

1. Family members are to be regarded as one choice;

2. Loved ones and friends are to be regarded as one choice;

3. Pets, regardless of their species and number, are also to be regarded as one choice.

That's three on your list, what are the other seventeen?

Just in case you are struggling to put pen to paper, reflect on the following as this might just help focus your thinking.

- What would you save in the event of a disaster such as a fire or a flood?

- What would you/do you hide from potential thieves?

- If you were taken into prison what would you want to safeguard?

- If you were forced to live under a different political régime that is very different from that which you know, what would be most important to you?

- Bad things happen to people all the time in our world. What if they were to happen to you?

Here's my list:
1. Family – that includes the people I love most of all in the world.
2. Friends – a life without friends would be empty.
3. My happy box, which contains all sorts of daft-looking oddments and souvenirs but they are important to me.
4. Photographs – there are many albums detailing different experiences and people in my life.
5. My privacy – I hold it dear.
6. My right to speak out and voice my opinion.
7. My own space and the freedom to choose to be where I want to be.
8. My books – I have many.
9. My CD collection from ABBA to Zeppelin.
10. My computer and all my memory sticks (that may count as two).
11. My lovely car – it's not brilliant but it gets me about.
12. Good food and wine – I do love both.
13. My job and my role as a senior lecturer, and contact with students.
14. My allotment and all the fruit and vegetables it produces.
15. My mobile phone.
16. The beautiful jewellery that people have bought me over the years.
17. My independence.

18. My knowledge of the world and my mental capacity (that's two really).
19. Making my own decisions about how I live.
20. My physical health.

Creating that list, knowing that it would be up for public view, was no easy task, even though I am experienced in helping others to do the same. Perhaps you struggled or maybe you found it easy. Does your list go beyond twenty items? Can you compare your list with other people's lists? Are they similar in any way?

My guess is that there are many things similar within our lists but, regardless of similarities or differences, the most important thing is that the list represents what is important to you and can be seen as a marker of who you are and what you hold dear. Our personality is often portrayed by the things we hold dear. (If you are interested in finding out a little about yourself and your personality you might wish to follow this link and take the adapted Myers–Briggs Personality Test: www.humanmetrics.com/cgi-win/jtypes2.asp).

## UNDERSTANDING OURSELVES AND OTHER PEOPLE

Psychology can teach us a great deal about ourselves and about other people and, as a person working in the care services, it is important that you understand some of the basic tenets of psychological study. *Chapter 2* will have helped you to think about how you have developed as a person and it emphasises the importance of self-awareness. Understanding yourself and how you prefer to be with others will provide you with valuable information about your personal communication style and why you get on well with some people and not others. Adapting our responses to individuals can help the communication process to flow more easily.

Psychology can also be useful in helping us understand the impact our self-esteem has upon us as individuals and, in particular, the way in which self-esteem is important to psychological health. How we feel about ourselves and what we hold dear is directly affected by changes in our health status. Gross and Kinson (2007) discuss the development of the self-concept and offer examples of how changes to our physical bodies can impact on our perception of self and consequently alter our behaviour. Indeed, the whole text is worthy of a read.

**REFLECTION** 6.2

I want you now to think about a person that you have had experience of working with or being with who has had to be admitted into care: health care as an emergency, or social care as a planned event as a consequence of alterations in their physical or psychological health.

REFLECTION · 6.2 CONT'D

Using your skills of self-awareness and empathy, imagine what it must have been like to be that person.

What was the response from the care agencies involved?

If you found yourself in a similar situation, how would you feel?

If you were that person and had that experience of being admitted into care, how many things on the list that you previously generated do you think would still be immediately available to you? Work systematically through your list of twenty things and score out those that would not be available. Then erase components of those things that perhaps may be available but only in small measures. For example, your family and friends whose access to you is likely to be limited due to visiting rules. You can't have all your photos with you but you could have a snapshot in your purse/wallet. It's all about compromise. On admission into care it is likely that you would be advised about the safe-keeping of valuables and you would be asked to turn off your mobile phone. It is more than likely that your privacy would be seriously invaded with questioning and possible examination and your right to be free to determine your own daily activities would be, in the first instance, severely curtailed. Your car would be left at home as parking is always expensive and difficult, and you certainly would not have your own bed or chair. Everything around you would be unfamiliar.

Go through your list and share your thoughts with a friend, fellow student or your teacher or mentor and see what is left on that list as a result of being admitted into care. It is likely that you will strike out the majority of those things you listed.

I always find this a sobering thing to do but it is a really useful exercise to undertake because it gives us an insight into what people experience when they are taken from their own surroundings, either because they are too ill or just too frail to take care of themselves. The admission into care is often not a positive experience.

The people who are in need of either health or social care lose so much in accepting the care that they need. The arguments as to whether it is 'for the best' fade in comparison with what a person has to give up in relation to their independence and freedom 'to be'. Nicholson-Perry and Burgess (2002) discuss the ways in which people who suffer serious illness have to adapt, both psychologically and socially, as their health status changes. With illness comes a personal change of perception of who we are, and our lifestyle and relationships all have to change too. When a person is faced with so much loss, the feelings of the Child ego state can be overwhelming. Despair, fear, anger, abandonment, grief, resentment and bitterness are, sadly, common experiences of those admitted into care.

# BLOCKS AND BARRIERS TO EFFECTIVE COMMUNICATION

There are times when it is more difficult to communicate effectively either because of what is happening around you or because of what is happening within you or the person that you are trying to communicate with.

**WRITING ACTIVITY** 6.1

- Make a list of all the factors that make listening difficult. You should consider both external and internal factors.
- Reflect on which are obvious and easily noticed and which are more difficult to pick up on.

Your lists might look something like this:

**Internal**
- Difference in culture and values
- Negative feelings towards the client
- Trying to hypothesise about what's *really* going on
- Working out what you're going to say next
- Getting upset / annoyed about what the client is saying
- Trying to find solutions
- Feelings of inadequacy
- Difficulties in your life
- Feeling unsafe

**External**
- Tiredness
- Hunger
- Feeling ill
- Noise
- Inappropriate environment
- Client has complex needs
- Client does not speak English
- Client is deaf / hearing impaired

## How to deal with blocks and barriers

The Shannon and Weaver Model shown in *Figure 1.1* describes the things that impact on communication as 'noise' which can be literal noise or some other kind of internal or external noise which can act as a barrier. The most important way for you to avoid a barrier to communication is to be aware of your own 'stuff', be it internal or external, so that you can avoid responding to the person you are supporting from your own frame of reference.

*Chapter 3* has already dealt with the external blocks that arise because of cultural or language barriers. When the block is external like noise, hunger, tiredness or illness you have to be aware and prepared to negotiate that block in a caring and sensitive way. If there is too much noise, you can ask the person to come somewhere quieter so that you can talk and listen properly. It's never advisable to try to talk above a noise. As already mentioned in *Chapter 2*, you must be responsible for your own physical wellbeing so that if you are tired, hungry or ill you deal with it and avoid situations where you will not be able to concentrate or to listen properly. If you have to make decisions based on the communication that you have with others, it is particularly important that you do not allow barriers to get in the way.

If the blocks are internal and you find that you are not able to listen effectively, you need to be self-aware enough to notice what is going on for you and what might be going on for the other person. If you look back at the example of a care home worker using the CLT Reflective Model, you will see how she was able to notice the 'noise' that was blocking her communication with Mr C's son. She realised that if she had used active listening skills she would have avoided being rude and she might have enabled Mr C's son to explore his anxiety and his worries for his Dad. She realised that she needed to show him empathy even when she didn't agree with him. She used her insight to become more aware of Mr C and his son's frames of reference and so the barrier was more likely to fall away. If the barrier is due to your emotional overload you need to be able to recognise your limitations. Sometimes it can be hard to carry around someone else's pain or anxiety or anger or sadness. *Chapter 2* suggested ways that you could manage situations like that.

## DEALING WITH DIFFICULT PEOPLE

Sometimes there is a block because the person that you are trying to communicate with is really difficult and determined to create barriers, refusing to let you in. Good communication is described by Burnard (1989) as the bedrock of good care but sometimes even good communication and interpersonal skills cannot easily manage the situation, particularly when emotions are high. People are not rational all of the time. When faced with fear and uncertainty they respond angrily and this can create difficult situations which if not defused adequately can lead to aggressive action.

**READING ACTIVITY** 6.1

Difficult people are all around us. The category of difficult people may even include you! The Institute of Management Excellence has an online newsletter available at www.itstime.com/. This website offers some really interesting links and explores how to deal with difficult people in the workplace through the use of Personality Dragons.

The dragons include:
* greed
* impatience
* arrogance
* stubbornness
* self-deprecation
* martyrdom
* self-determination.

These are interesting takes on the different sorts of personalities that we find ourselves working with and the website offers tried-and-tested solutions for given sets of circumstances. The Institute of Management Excellence offers some very sensible advice about how to manage emotionally-fuelled conflict and in summary suggests the following.
* Question your own defensiveness. Why are you upset by this situation? Remember defensiveness often fuels anger, leading to a worse situation.
* Stay focused in an irrational attack. See it as a gift that you do not have to accept. It is not personal.
* Calmly ask the person what they are upset about and accept that there is some kernel of truth in their complaint.
* Ask for feedback. Being on their side will enable you to defuse the situation more quickly.
* Don't try to win the fight – it is best to go for a win–win situation.
* Listen carefully and ask questions to elicit the nature of the complaint.
* Appreciate and don't blame.

When conflict occurs it is a problem for all those concerned and it needs to be dealt with carefully. Understanding what motivates people and fuels their emotions will help to pull the situation back to something that can be agreed upon and worked on jointly. In circumstances such as these using leverage is a good strategy. For example, 'If you agree to come with me now I'll sort out an appointment with your social worker and we'll see if we can sort something out'.

**REFLECTION** 6.3

Sometimes people's views can present you with specific dilemmas. The British Medical Journal published an article entitled *Managing patients who express racist views* (Baraitser, 2006). This article presents a dilemma and asks four professionals to give their views on the best way to handle the following situation:

*You are a junior doctor working in a family planning clinic. A patient of yours needs referral to one of several senior doctors who work in your organisation for a complicated intrauterine device fitting. You recommend a colleague who has expertise*

**REFLECTION** 6.3 CONT'D

*in this field and the patient agrees to be referred. However, when you mention the name of the doctor, the patient realises she might be from an ethnic minority and requests a referral to someone else. What should you do?*

You can find this article at: http://jfprhc.bmj.com/content/32/1/47

Before you read it reflect on what you would do in a similar situation. Discuss the dilemma with your colleagues or fellow students. When you have had this discussion, read the article and reflect on what the four professionals had to say.

If your strategies for dealing with difficult people fail, it is important to remember that even if other people do not behave or respond differently, you can. Self-awareness and a willingness to learn are essential requirements to developing your own skill but when the situation involves strong emotions in the people you are caring for or working with, effective communication and interpersonal skills are crucial.

Emotions such as anger, despair, panic, love or hate can lead to atypical and unpredictable behaviour and this unpredictability then produces strong emotions in others. If a person that you are trying to support is extremely angry then it is very difficult not to act instinctively and either retreat or fight back. Both of these responses are natural but unprofessional. Panic can lead to poor judgement and impaired skills.

The most important thing to remember is to seek help if you find you are out of your depth. There are no medals available for people who attempt to deal with situations that they cannot handle and the rule of thumb is that if the situation scares you tell the person that you can't deal with that situation and that you have to leave to get someone else to help them. Most people when angry are operating from their Child ego state and are out of control. Being faced by someone who tells them that they cannot handle this situation is often enough to jolt them back to a temporary thinking state as they realise the impact they are having on other people.

In *Figure 6.1* the Angry Child ego state on the left is verbally abusing the helper's Child ego state on the right. This other person's angry Child ego state is fuelled to some extent internally via the person's Parent ego state. The Critical Parent is conveying messages such as 'how dare they do this to me, I don't need to tolerate this, tell them just what you think of them right now.' The Adult ego state is not currently being accessed so there is very little thinking taking place.

Although the helper's Child ego state is naturally ready to respond to this person's anger by being defensive or by being angry back, they do not have to accept this interaction. They can instead choose to use rationality and respond from their Adult ego state, pitching to transact with the Adult ego state of the other person.

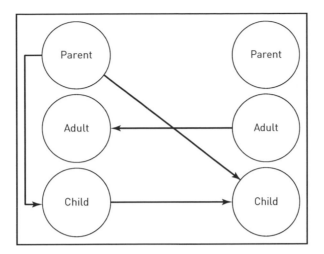

**Figure 6.1** *Transactional Analysis of dealing with a difficult person.*

For example, a safe Adult ego state response could be, 'you seem to be very upset and you do have a serious complaint to make but I am not really equipped to deal with this. Can you please wait here and I will get someone who can help you'. The other person's Adult ego state is being addressed in this transaction, resulting in a momentary defusion of the situation and the Critical Parent ego state then needs to think and respond, probably with something like, 'yes, I do have a serious complaint to make, you had better go get somebody who can sort it out'. This will give you sufficient time to move away and seek help.

Genuine anger bursts out and results in tears as the emotion is burned out. The skilled communicator can stay with that person until the tears come and the emotional response begins to calm down. Those who stay angry are likely to be psychologically disturbed and pose a risk for others, and steps to safeguard others may need to be taken. When someone is in a very angry state it is important that you stay calm and deal with the situation, especially if you are the only one available at that time.

The following guidelines are useful if you find yourself in a situation where someone is angry and aggressive:

## Verbal de-escalation
- Use a one-to-one approach
- Use the individual's name
- Ask open questions
- Enquire about the reason for the anger
- Don't be defensive even when abuse is directed at you
- Ask questions about facts rather than feelings

- Answer informational questions but avoid abusive ones
- Show concern and empathy, use active listening skills
- Acknowledge their grievances, concerns and frustrations but don't interpret or analyse their feelings
- Use slow clear speech
- Keep your volume and tone quiet and calm
- Don't patronise them, be respectful
- Give choices where appropriate.

## Non-verbal de-escalation

- Maintain limited eye contact and a neutral facial expression
- Have open body language and minimise the gestures you use
- Allow greater body space than normal
- Consider the position of your body, be at the same eye level as the person, face them and ensure that you have clear access to the exit
- Minimise your movement, stay as still as possible
- Appear calm, self-controlled and confident without being dismissive or overbearing.

---

**ACTIVITY**

Read these statements and think about how they would be heard by someone who is really angry:

- Please don't behave like this, I'm only trying to help
- If you don't stop that immediately, you'll be in big trouble
- Alan, I can see that you are angry. Shall I give you some space or would you like to sit down and we can talk about what's bothering you?

---

## WORKING IN ORGANISATIONS AND COMMUNICATING WITH OTHERS

As shown in *Chapters 2* and *5*, we need to listen to ourselves, those in our care and those who can give us feedback about our performance, but we also need to communicate with and listen to those with whom we work in partnership. Carnwell and Buchanan (2005) make clear the point that in recognising the needs of those we care for we must also recognise the role of others in providing for people's needs. There is a danger within service provision to see only the care that we ourselves can offer and ignore what other agencies and professionals can provide. Effective care relies on us being able to work in partnership, and being able to communicate with people from other agencies ensures that those we care for receive the best possible care.

Carnwell and Buchanan (2005) outline the dangers of professional groups working in isolation. Specialisation and professionalism have led us to a situation where subject-specific language can be difficult to understand and often contributes to a breakdown in communication between agencies and organisations. It is recognised that understanding the role of others will help in ensuring seamless working with people. Networking and joined-up thinking are now at the centre of providing effective care, and professional and volunteer groups need to find new ways of communicating and working in partnership. Jelphs (2006) outlines what she believes to be the key areas for organisations, teams and individuals to consider.

- How to develop and implement a meaningful communication strategy;
- How the strategy links to other strategic policies and procedures;
- How information is shared between staff;
- The ability of staff to access communication systems;
- How information is shared between patients and service users;
- How to develop information that is empowering and enabling for staff and service users;
- How to manage the grapevine;
- How to manage the media.

These are all big issues to consider. Sharing information requires a language that all can understand and developing that level of understanding requires everyone involved to be proactive and open to change.

## CODES OF PRACTICE

As previously discussed, poor communication is often at the centre of complaints that people make against the NHS, and staff attitude in particular is one of the main reasons for complaint. The NHS is a massive organisation and the communication systems are many, with each one tailored to meet the need for recording and sharing information. The NHS Records Management Code of Practice is available online at: www.gov.uk/government/publications/records-management-nhs-code-of-practice. This website provides a great deal of material to read with regard to communication, and the links there are very useful, covering all aspects of modes and channels of communication that were discussed in *Chapter 1*. Organisations that seek to help people must have criteria that they use to guide the practice of those who work for them. Codes of practice offer criteria that can be used to review your own personal performance as a person working in the helping professions and may also be used by your employers to judge your practice and your ability.

READING ACTIVITY   6.2

Which code of practice do you use to review your performance? The following websites are recommended to you, subject to your specific role:

**www.nmc-uk.org** for nurses and midwives;

**www.skillsforcare.com** for the General Social Care Council (GSCC) codes of practice.

## THE WRITTEN WORD

Each of these codes of conduct makes reference to communication and record-keeping. Working with people will require you to take part in recording detail. Being able to maintain clear and accurate records will be part of your role. Record-keeping is an integral part of all healthcare practice and is essential to the provision of safe, effective care. The level of supervision that you receive will be subject to your role and position within the organisation but there may come a time when you are responsible for writing and maintaining official records. The kinds of writing that we are required to do at work will include:

- telephone messages
- patient notes
- case reviews
- notes for patients
- messages in the handover book
- emails
- text messages.

In the interests of patient safety and in our increasingly litigious society, it is of great importance that the records we keep are meticulous. They are an important means of communication between staff and agencies and are available to the individual at their request. Communication, whether verbal or written, is about delivering a message and when it is written there is no non-verbal information, so it needs to be done clearly and unambiguously. Patients or any other service user can request copies of their notes so care must be taken with how things are expressed.

Records were previously kept mainly in paper form but, with the development of technology, they are increasingly being kept in electronic form. It is important to remember that the contents and quality of these records will have consequences for those being cared for and for you as the carer. They are legal documents that may be called for scrutiny at any time. As such, records should be

- accurate in their detail;
- concise and appropriate;

- contemporaneous (meaning up-to-date);
- objective and non-judgemental – there is no room for subjective material;
- legible – others must be able to read them;
- kept safe and with confidentiality maintained;
- signed and dated by the person who has written them.

The Data Protection Act (1998) is available online at www.legislation.gov.uk/ukpga/1998/29/contents and details the legal principles that underpin the regulation of the processing of information relating to people. You should familiarise yourself with these details to protect yourself and the people whom you work with.

# TELEPHONE

How many times have you tried to communicate with an organisation by phone and been left feeling really frustrated? You may recall from *Chapter 3* that only 7% of the communication that takes place normally is via the words used, so it is no wonder that the telephone is so difficult to use and so fraught with problems. If you look back to the discussion regarding communication models, the Transmission Model was designed specifically to help overcome difficulties experienced in telecommunication. Many organisations now give training on customer care and telephone technique and this has come about as a response to the many complaints received. It is important that you seek the advice and training of your employer but the following principles will certainly help you avoid running into difficulty when answering the phone.

- Clearly state the name of the organisation / agency or place of work.
- State your name and your position.
- Ask how you can help.

For example:

- Ward 10 Redwood hospital, Susan Jones, student nurse, can I help you? or…
- Ashleigh Wood Care Home, Gillian Smith, receptionist, can I help? or…
- Northwood Rehabilitation Unit, Tom Brown, care assistant, can I help?

You need to find the most comfortable way of introducing yourself, your status and your place of work. You may wish to say 'hello' or 'good afternoon' and that preference is up to you but the principle here is that when a person calls they need to know they have the right telephone number and to whom they are speaking. A good reply is one that gives those details, one that sounds professional and calm and one that is welcoming of the telephone call. If you have stated those things clearly it is likely that the caller will then respond positively, e.g. 'Yes, this is Doctor Mead, can I speak to …'

Don't just say 'hello' as it leaves the caller struggling as to what to say next and it is unprofessional. Even if you have access to a telephone that gives you the caller's identity, never assume it is them as other people may be using their phone.

Also be aware that detail should not be given over the phone that is confidential. If in doubt, seek advice from your mentor or manager.

## EMAIL AND TEXT

Email has been used as a way of communicating within and between organisations for many years. It saves time, it is auditable and it can be incredibly effective, but it is also one of the most frustrating, mainly because of the number of unnecessary emails that are sent. Round robins and circulars may raise the odd smile but they clutter up your in tray and distract the eye from what may be important, and it is more than likely that your organisation would frown upon the system being used in such a way. Don't use the email for anything it is not intended to be used for. Check your employer's policies for email use and do not fall foul of it as your job could be at stake.

Texting and emailing via mobile phone is also used increasingly, depending on organisations' individual policies. You should only use a work mobile phone for work calls, texts or emails; using your personal number or email address blurs the boundaries between professional and personal and could lead to unintentional mistakes if you end up sending group texts or emails. In addition and most importantly, there are huge implications of data protection when the use of mobile phones involves working with personal data. In my work as a counsellor I almost always use text to contact and be contacted by my clients to set up, change or cancel appointments but their names in my contacts list are disguised and no personal information is used. The majority of texts are simple appointment times or changes but I do delete the texts straight away once my diary is updated. If a client texts me anything else, I put any important information in my notes which are kept securely. I also ensure that I write texts in a formal way. If you were brought up with emails, texts and social media as a natural form of communication you might be used to using a particular kind of written communication which includes abbreviations, slang and, more recently, creative punctuation and little symbols called emoticons. In professional contexts, emails and texts should be in standard English with correct spelling, grammar and punctuation.

There are certain principles that you should be aware of when using email or text and attending to the following will help to prevent misinterpretation and keep the message reasonably intact.

- Is email/text the best mode of communication to use?
- Should you be sending this detail via email/text and is it confidential?
- To whom are you sending it and what do you want them to do with it?
- If you are using your employer's computer system you must attend to their protocols.
- Address the email carefully.
- Flag up if you want a reply, receipt or confirmation of reading.

- Be polite and use 'please' and 'thank you' as appropriate.
- Check the tone of the message.
- Try to be as concise and professional as you can.
- NEVER USE UPPERCASE, AS IT LOOKS AS IF YOU ARE SHOUTING.
- Check the spelling and the grammar before sending the email/text.
- Send it only to the people who need to receive it.

The ease of sending messages via email makes it an attractive option but remember that when messages are sent and received electronically you do not have that opportunity to talk face-to-face with that person, and there is a danger that priorities will be missed and information misinterpreted. You will not be able to see the receiver's reaction nor judge how the email was received. The very essence of email suggests that a quick response is required, but it is important that you take your time in wording the email and detailing the response time to the receiver. Short turnaround times may result in quick decisions that have not been fully thought through.

## SOCIAL MEDIA

Since the start of the 21st century, communication via social media such as Facebook, Twitter, LinkedIn and other sites which I have probably not heard of, has created new options for extending and enhancing communication. However, as the number and use of these new channels of communication increase, so does the potential for mistakes and misuse. Even experienced users of social media and technology can get caught out. Hardly a week goes by without the media reporting something that some high profile person has tweeted which has got them into trouble of one kind or another.

Maintaining professional boundaries in all forms of communication is vital to maintaining trust and professional relationships. The use of social networking in professional settings creates challenges for managing risks for both individuals and organisational reputations alike, but it can also open up communication and provide opportunities for learning and development. The NHS Social Media Toolkit states: "In the NHS, the use of social media has evolved from communications teams tweeting press releases to staff and leaders at all levels taking part in spontaneous and structured conversations across multiple platforms." This suggests that there are more and more opportunities for NHS staff to engage in discussions on social media and the same is true of social care settings. Increasingly organisations such as the NHS and social care providers are thinking about how to use the services and websites that staff are already familiar with in their personal lives to enhance and benefit their professional lives (Skills for Care, 2013). If you are using social media within your professional setting you should adhere to the Code of Conduct of that setting and follow the guidelines for all written communication given above. In addition and very importantly you must always consider confidentiality and safeguarding when talking or writing about work issues.

> **CHAPTER SUMMARY**
>
> ### Seven key points to take away from Chapter 6:
>
> - Big life transitions like leaving home and going into a care setting can have a huge and potentially devastating impact on people's lives, their self-esteem and their emotional wellbeing.
>
> - Our self-awareness is particularly important when there are blocks and barriers to effective communication.
>
> - When we have to deal with difficult people and manage strong emotions we must continue to use our skills of empathy, acceptance, and self-awareness rather than retreat or act defensively.
>
> - Working with other agencies and organisations is an essential part of joined-up care and service provision.
>
> - Codes of practice provide information and guidelines on how to work ethically and keep the service users' needs at the forefront of your mind.
>
> - Written communication and record-keeping are a key part of health and social care provision.
>
> - All written communication must stay within professional boundaries.

## SUGGESTED READING

Carnwell and Buchanan's *Effective Practice in Health and Social Care* (2005) is a useful text to help you understand some of the challenges that the caring services currently face and is well worth a read.

## REFERENCES

Baraitser, P. (2006) Managing patients who express racist views. *The Journal of Family Planning and Reproductive Healthcare*. **32:1**, pp 47–48. Available at: http://jfprhc.bmj.com/content/32/1/47 (accessed 13 February 2015).

Burnard, P. (1989) *Teaching Interpersonal Skills. A handbook of experiential learning for health professionals*. London: Chapman and Hall.

Carnwell, R. and Buchanan, J. (eds) (2005) *Effective Practice in Health and Social Care*. Milton Keynes: Open University Press.

Challem, J. (2007) 'Theanine. The calm in your tea'. *Better Nutrition*, **69(6) 32:** pp. 34–35.

Gross, R. and Kinson, N. (2007) *Psychology for Nurses and Allied Health Professionals*. London: Hodder Arnold.

Jelphs, K. (2006) Communication: soft skill, hard impact? *Clinician in Management*, **14:** pp. 33–37.

NHS Employers (2014) A Social Media Toolkit for the NHS. Available at: www. nhsemployers.org/~/media/Employers/Publications/NHS_Social_Media_ Toolkit_%20Introduction_and_Process.pdf (accessed 9 February 2015).

Skills for Care (2013) Learning technologies in social care. Available at: www. skillsforcare.org.uk/document-library/qualifications-and-apprenticeships/ learning-technology/learningtechnologiesinsocialcare-aguideforemployers.pdf (accessed 13 February 2015).

# 07

# CASE STUDY

This chapter uses a case study to bring together and review the ideas, principles and details that have been discussed in previous chapters with regard to communication and interpersonal skills. The case study illustrates an elderly person's perception of being admitted into care and shows the importance of communication throughout that process. This is just one person's story and the consent of the gentleman to whom this happened has been sought and gained. Bill Jones, whose name has been changed to protect his identity, has read the chapter and confirms the content. Seeking consent is described by Bradshaw and Merriman (2007) as a "fundamental part of a therapeutic relationship" and they comment that "seeking consent is a process and not just a one-off event". Bill hopes that his story will go some way to helping others see what it is like to be admitted into care and that it will help improve the communication skills of carers, particularly in those first few weeks that he described as being a particularly horrible time for him.

## CASE STUDY:

### An experience of care

Bill is an elderly gentleman who has lived alone for many years following the death of his wife. He has no children but he was supported by good friends and neighbours who, over the years, took on many responsibilities to help ensure that Bill was safe and cared for. He was fiercely independent and had learned many new skills as he adjusted to living on his own but, as the years unfolded, his health deteriorated and arthritis took its toll on his mobility and his ability to care for himself.

Like many elderly people he experienced several falls in the house and outside in his beloved garden, causing himself physical damage and resulting in him being fearful of being on his own. He had several emergency admissions to the local A&E department and, following a request for a social need assessment, arrangements were made for him to be supported at home. Several appliances were delivered to help with his daily activities – grab bars were situated around the house to help him mobilise and a commode was installed in his bedroom. He agreed to receive daily visits from a care agency who offered support with meals and help with personal and daily living activities. Although this meant Bill had to compromise on how he chose to live, he did adjust and the system worked reasonably well for some months.

Bradshaw and Merriman (2007) outline useful principles in communicating with the older person, paying particular regard to dignity, privacy and comfort. It would be true to say that all those people who served Bill in his own home were respectful of his personal space, paid regard to the normal protocols expected when entering someone's home and treated him as a fellow human being. There was a great deal of humour used by the workmen who fitted the grab bars and the delivery of the commode resulted in all the 'throne jokes' you can think of. This certainly helped to ease what was an uncomfortable situation for Bill. The skill of these people was to treat Bill as an equal and it worked. They all referred to him as Mr Jones and took no liberties in assuming the right to use his first name. The carers who came to the house soon established good rapport with him by being professional and respectful in helping him to meet his own needs.

In your role as a carer it is extremely important to maintain that professional attitude towards those you work with, and you need to check all the time that your approach is acceptable to them. I am allowed to call Bill by his first name but I had known him for five years before he invited me to call him Bill. Friendship is not to be assumed, particularly when you are working as a professional, and calling older people by their first name without being invited to do so is often viewed by the older person as being forward and impolite.

> Bill was determined to stay at home and the support system seemed to be working well but, while the neighbour who would normally call in at lunchtime was away on holiday, the late-afternoon carer arrived to find Bill on the floor where he had been for several hours, nursing a damaged forehead and a swollen wrist. He was in a poor condition, chilled to the bone, confused and unable to stand and, following a trip to the A&E department, he was admitted into residential care.
>
> It is reported that on admission into care he was confused, shouting loudly, demanding to be taken back home and was very rude to the people who tried to approach him. It was the ambulance driver who transferred Bill to the residential unit from the hospital who eventually calmed him down to the point that he agreed to stay, at least for the time being.

This was a major life event for Bill to adjust to. What he deemed to be safe was not acceptable to the care service who had been invited in to help him at home. Bill was very angry that his independence was, as he describes it, 'being taken away from me'. He saw his life being taken apart and there was nothing that he could do to stop it. Had he the ability to walk, he would have walked away but he was almost immobile, bruised and battered from his fall and unable to cope alone. There was no family to rescue him and take him home, there was a lot of anger and resentment on his part and he blamed all the people around him for letting him down, even those who were trying to help.

Bill was responding to what was happening to him from his Child ego state. He had all sorts of misconceptions about what happened to people when they were admitted into care and, as he said to me, 'I have never felt so helpless in all my life. I wanted to hit out at them but I couldn't even do that'.

**READING ACTIVITY** 7.1

We should stop here for a moment and consider the process of taking someone like Bill into care. There are several frameworks that offer guidance and advice in setting care standards for the elderly, in particular The National Service Framework for Older People (2001). This is available online at:

www.gov.uk/government/uploads/system/uploads/attachment_data/file/198033/ National_Service_Framework_for_Older_People.pdf

Another useful area to review is that of the Human Rights Act 1998. This is available online at www.legislation.gov.uk/ukpga/1998/42/contents. You will find many useful links there to follow as you require. You may wish to supplement your reading with other texts in this series with regard to values and ethical dilemmas.

For those working with children and families I recommend a visit to the following website: www.legislation.gov.uk/ukpga/2004/31/contents

This will provide many links to legislative frameworks including the Children Act 2004 and other links concerning children and young people.

Taking anyone into any form of care is a major step, whether that care is planned or unplanned, scheduled or unscheduled, involves hospitalisation or any form of residential care. Consent must be sought whether the person is young or old and this can be achieved only by using good communication skills. Nicholson-Perry and Burgess (2002) comment that "good communication empowers people to make informed choices that are right for them as individuals". Sometimes those choices are limited, as in the case of Bill who knew he had no alternative choices available to him at that time and had to accept the place that was found for him, albeit on a temporary basis. It was the responsibility of those around him to help him, to reassure him and to give him hope for the future. The way to do that is through good communication skills and proactively using counselling skills to help the person in crisis.

Bill had an individual room at the end of a very long corridor, all very uniform in design, with lots of posters and information around detailing fire exits and directions to various locations. His room had an en suite bathroom facility, his meals were ready cooked and served to him either within the dining room or in his own room, there was a doctor on call and care staff to assist him in everything he needed. It sounds idyllic but that is not how Bill saw it.

When a friend visited she found he was dressed in someone else's pyjamas and his clothes were still in his suitcase. They had been left there because they were not labelled and there was a fear they would be lost. A congealed meal lay cold on a tray on his bed, which was too short for his tall frame, and he had only one pillow, which was too soft to support his aching neck. He had not been allowed to walk alone for fear of another fall and he had to rely on the staff attending to him for his every need. One of the young women carers even called him Mr Billy. He was not impressed. His complaints to his friend would fill many pages but all she could do at that point was to listen as his Child ego state poured out all the injustices to which he felt he had been subjected. He was angry, he was scared about the future and he cried.

## Dealing with anger

Bill's friend took a very rational approach to the complaints that she heard and, operating in her Adult ego state, she acted as his advocate. She asked many direct questions of those who were responsible for caring for him, taking care to raise his complaints and concerns in a rational enquiring manner. The majority of the responses to the questions asked appeared to be defensive and the nurses and carers alike were often very patronising, causing ill feeling and distrust. Thomas (2003) shows that the combination of time constraints and high workloads often leaves nurses feeling defensive and responding to complaints in a defensive manner. Thomas goes on to outline the way in which defensiveness can add to the already emotional situation and result in anger. Anger and emotional outbursts are commonplace in care settings. Where else would you find such vulnerable people? It is no surprise that anger is the most common emotion expressed.

As people working in health and social care facilities it is important to appreciate the role of anger in everyday living. Rather than viewing it as something to be feared, you need to explore what underpins and motivates anger and identify the ways in which you can harness the energy spent through anger, and use that energy elsewhere. Anger serves a really important function in life. It helps us cope with stress and to express our feelings. Anger and the expression of anger are influenced by our coping strategies, and our feelings of being out of control and vulnerable are often expressed as anger, which is often directed at those around us.

Whether those around us deserve that anger is another issue but, for now, we will accept that anger is a common reaction to difficult circumstances and that none of us is rational all of the time. Working in a helping capacity you need to develop a strategy for coping with the expression of highly charged emotions by those receiving care and also to cope with the emotions of the families who observe the care process and also feel helpless. We have looked at dealing with strong emotions in *Chapter 5*.

Staff cited Bill's mild confusion to explain many of his complaints, which made him feel even angrier and led to many verbal outbursts. This resulted in staff finding him difficult to communicate with and therefore withdrawing from him. Over a period of time Bill's anger turned to helplessness and he became increasingly unhappy and uncommunicative, which was interpreted as a decline in his condition. Despite an attempt to improve relationships and get people communicating with one another it was eventually agreed that the placement was not suitable and Bill, with the support and help of his friends and neighbours, set about finding somewhere that he would be happy to spend the rest of his days.

This was a man whose life was being diminished in a way that he found unacceptable. He felt as if he had been locked away, and the way of living in this particular establishment encroached upon all the things he held dear. His privacy, his independence, his comfort, his freedom were all affected by things that were out of his direct control, and his day was determined by other people, many of whom he had no relationship with at all even after several weeks of living there. The breakdown in communication was unfortunate and indicated a need for communication training among the staff.

Jelphs (2006) discusses the way in which the very mention of communication skills to health care professionals causes raised eyebrows. She states that "something as fundamental as communication is seen as a soft skill" and goes on to comment that "communication is the skill that can possibly have the greatest impact on effective health care delivery". Communication and active listening skills can be learned and used by all helpers to help prevent breakdown in care and facilitate a positive care experience.

A new care home was found and the experience of being admitted into the new establishment was very different. First and foremost Bill had a say in where it was he should go. He visited several places before he made his choice. The transfer was planned and he saw his room before accepting it to be his. He negotiated with care staff about what he could have brought from home and this included a writing bureau, many papers and files detailing important information regarding his finances and history, his own TV and video recorder, his own duvet, pillows and bedding, several pictures, photographs, ornaments and, most important, his electric buggy and his pipe. He was invited to complete a questionnaire about his life and daily living activities, an assessment of his ability to care for himself was undertaken with his permission and a temporary contract for care was agreed.

Bill thought this to be very important. He wanted to make sure the home suited his needs before finalising details and signing up for the long term. This process was accommodated easily with the managers of the care home, who agreed wholeheartedly that there should be a trial period before Bill had to make up his mind and take up permanent residence.

On his arrival at his new home Bill expressed many anxieties. What if he didn't like it, what about his house, what did he need to have immediately available to him, what about the cat, his newspapers and the mail, who would bring his things, etc.? He was welcomed personally by the manager of the unit and his things were treated with great reverence and respect. Staff arranged to have all his clothes and bedding labelled and arrangements were made for the safe transportation of his possessions. His key worker sat with him and recorded all his concerns and then helped him map out strategies for dealing with all of them, contacting friends and neighbours on his behalf.

Bill now has a new daily routine. He has a choice of meals and always eats at the table, apart from breakfast which he prefers in his own room. He has freedom of movement and his electric buggy has a parking place close to hand. He has a room with a door leading to the outside world where the gardens are splendid and he is free to roam during daytime hours. So he can go and smoke his pipe in the garden in peace. One of the carers supplied him with a bird guide book so that he could learn the names of the birds that visited the feeding table situated outside his window. He has a safety call button that he wears around his neck in case he is in need of urgent assistance, and he has at hand his own money and easy access to an expense account set up by his solicitor, who has Power of Attorney and is now overseeing his finances and the sale of his house.

There is a great deal of political debate about the payment of care bills in this country but I do not have room to discuss this here. The most important thing for Bill is that he had the opportunity to request the setting up of the legal process for Power of Attorney, as he recognised that his confusion is likely to increase as he grows older. Coming to this point of self-awareness was all part of the change process for Bill. Many people helped him through those difficult decisions and realisations by having Adult to Adult ego state conversations with him, finally arranging for him to meet with his nominated solicitor. Just because someone has episodes of confusion does not mean that Adult to Adult conversations are impossible. Avoiding difficult conversations that need to be held only makes things worse in the long run. If you adhere to the Rogerian principles outlined in *Chapter 5* you will get the best out of people and empower them to maintain a level of personal integrity.

Bill has commented that the difference between this unit and the first one is that the staff listen to him, pay him due regard and respect his wishes. If he needs more toothpaste it is collected, if his whisky runs out he can arrange for a new bottle to be purchased for him. He can wander around the gardens in his buggy and smoke his pipe out of doors. He can invite friends to lunch with 24 hours' notice and he has his own mobile phone with him to keep in contact with his friends when he chooses. There is a residents' committee with which he is involved and there are lots of activities that he can either observe or take part in. Bill is still frail and at times confused and very cantankerous but he accepts that he needs care and accepts the care on offer. The staff in this unit demonstrate a positive regard towards him. The overarching philosophy of this unit is that it is the person's home and it should be as comfortable as their previous home was. Everything is achievable with a little thought and application and the staff use the skills of empathy and show the ability to understand what it is like to be old and frail and in Bill's situation. They actively listen to him and communicate with him in a positive way. He has become a person again.

We hope that this case study has helped you to understand the vital importance of effective communication. We all need to reflect on our own communication and interpersonal skills as they are fundamental to being an effective practitioner in whatever field you choose to work in. We trust that you have enjoyed reading and working with this text and we wish you well with your studies.

## REFERENCES

Bradshaw, A. and Merriman, C. (2007) *Caring for the Older Person*. Chichester: Wiley.

Jelphs, K. (2006) Communication: soft skill, hard impact? *Clinician in Management*, **14:** pp. 33–37.

Nicholson-Perry, K. and Burgess, M. (2002) *Communication in Cancer Care*. Oxford: BPS Blackwell.

Thomas, S.P. (2003) Anger: the mismanaged emotion. *Dermatological Nursing*, **15(4):** pp. 351–358.

# INDEX

Locators in *italic* refer to figures/diagrams

abandonment feelings, 102
acceptance, unconditional, 38, 82–3, 96
acknowledgment of feelings, 87–8, 93
acronym, social grraacceess, 53
Action on Hearing Loss guidelines (2014), 57–8
active listening, 85–94, 96
activities to practise
    dealing with difficult people, 108
    listening to people, 79
adapted child ego state, 68, 75
admission into care, ix, 101–2, 117–23
adult ego state, 62, 65–7, *70, 71, 72*
    being admitted into care case study, 122
    dealing with difficult people, 106, *107*
anger
    being admitted into care, 102, 120–3
    blocks to effective communication, 104
    dealing with difficult people, 105, 106–8
    ego states, 62
    listening to people, 80, 81, 83, 86
applications, *see* practical applications
asylum seekers, 56, 79
attitudes, ego states, 65, 68, 68–9
automatic thoughts, 27
avoidance behaviour, 28
awareness of self, *see* self-awareness

barriers to effective communication, 103–4, 114
Beck, A. T., 27
behaviour
    core/6 Cs, 2
    cultural perspectives, 52
    ego states, 64, 65, 68
beliefs, internal impacts on the self, 23–7

benevolence (doing good), 24
bereavement, 78
Berne, E., viii, 61–2, 67, 69, 72, 75
blocks to effective communication, 103–4, 114
body language, 58, 108
    dealing with difficult people, 108
    intercultural communication, 52
    interpersonal communication, 41, *45,* 46, 48, 52, 58
    listening to people, 45, 85–7, 91, 93, 94
Borton, T., 31–2
Bowlby, J., 5

care, being admitted into, ix, 101–2, 117–23
care home worker, *see* residential care home example
care, 6 Cs, 2
case study, being admitted into care, ix, 117–23
CBT (cognitive behavioural therapy), 27
Census 2011 (Office for National Statistics), 55–6
change/transition
    being admitted into care, 118
    listening to people, 78, 81
    Transactional Analysis, 75
    trauma of, 102, 114
channels, models of communication, *11,* 12, *14,* 15–16
child ego state, 62, 67–9, *70, 71, 72,* 75, 102
    being admitted into care case study, 119
    dealing with difficult people, 106, *107*
Children's Workforce Development Council, 3, 5
class, socioeconomic, 53

closed questions, 90–1

clothes, non-verbal communication through, 46–7, 51, 58

CLT model (three-step reflective cycle), 32–5, *33*, 104

Code of Conduct, Nursing and Midwifery Council, 94

codes of practice, 109–10, 114; *see also* guidelines

cognitive/affective disorder, 27

cognitive behavioural therapy (CBT), 27; *see also* mindfulness-based cognitive therapy

cognitive constraints, cultural perspectives, 52

commitment, 6 Cs, 2

*Common Core of skills and knowledge* (Children's Workforce Development Council), 3, 5

*Common Induction Standards*, 3

communication, viii, 16–17
    appropriate methods, 9–10
    barriers, 103–4
    definitions, 3–8, 13
    further reading, 17–18
    importance, 1–3
    intrapersonal, viii, 19–20
    modes, *see* modes of communication 6 Cs, 2
    through listening, 77–80
    *see also* interpersonal communication; practical application

communications theory, 10–16, *11*, *14*

compassion, 2, 21, 23

*Compassion in Practice: Nursing Midwifery and Care Staff. Our Vision and Strategy*, 3

competence, 6 Cs, 2

complaints, patient, 46

complementary transactions, 69–70, *70*

compliance, patient, 46

confidentiality, patient, 94–5, 96

conflict, 105; *see also* dealing with difficult people

conscientiousness, 24, 26

consent, patient, 119

Core Competencies for Healthcare Support Workers and Adult Social Care Workers, 85

core values and behaviours, 6 Cs, 2

courage, 6 Cs, 2

covert transactions, 72, *72*

critical parent ego state, 64, 72, 75, 106, 107

crossed transactions, *71*, 71–2

Crowley, P., 5

cultural perspectives, 51–7, 58, 88, 103, 104

curiosity, three-step reflective cycle, 32, 33, *33*

Data Protection Act (1998), 111

deaf people, 57–8, 103

decoding, transactional model, *14*

de-escalation, dealing with difficult people, 108

defensiveness, 105, 114

definitions
    communication, 3–8, 13
    emotions/feelings, 87

despair, 102

destination, Shannon and Weaver transmission model, *11*, 12

development framework, Borton, 31–2

difficult people, dealing with, 104–8, *107*, 114

dignity, 43, 118

disability, living with, 78, 81, 87

discernment, 24

disgust, 48

diversity, core dimensions, 5

divorce, 78

dress, non-verbal communication through, 46–7, 51, 58

education, cultural perspectives, 53

ego states, Transactional Analysis, 62–9

elderly people
    cultural perspectives, 53
    listening to people, 78

email, ix, 9, 110, 112–13

embarrassment, 43

emotional constraints, cultural perspectives, 52

emotional exhaustion, 20, 21; *see also* tiredness

*Emotional Intelligence* (Goleman), 27

emotions
    active listening, 87
    facial expressions, 48
    managing, 86, 106, 114, 120–3
    *see also* anger

empathic understanding, 38

empathy, 23
    being admitted into care example, 102
    dealing with difficult people, 114
    listening to people, 80–1, 85, 87, 88, 95

environmental communication, 49–51, 58

Equality Act (2010), 56

equality, core dimensions, 5

Ethical Framework for Good Practice in
        Counselling and Psychotherapy (2007),
        94
ethics
    codes of practice, 109–10, 114
    values, 5
ethnicity, 53; *see also* cultural perspectives
exhaustion, *see* tiredness
external impacts on the self
    barriers to effective communication,
        103
    self-awareness, 20–3
eye contact, 48, 51, 52, 86, 108

Facebook, 113
facial expressions, 48, 51, 108
fear, 44
    being admitted into care example,
        102, 117, 120
    facial expressions, 48
    listening to people, 80, 81, 88
feedback
    dealing with difficult people, 105
    three-step reflective cycle, 33, *33*, 34
feelings, acknowledging, 87–8, 93
first impressions, 40–1, 43
football red card, 6–7
Foss, K. A., 6
frameworks for theories of communication,
        10–11
Francis Report (Mid Staffordshire NHS
        Foundation Trust, 2013), 2
free child ego state, 68
French speaking example, negative thinking,
        27–8

gender, cultural perspectives, 53
genuineness, 38, 83–4, 95, 96
gesture, 47–8, 51, 58
    dealing with difficult people, 108
    intercultural communication, 52
    Parent ego state, 64
Goleman, D., 27
greetings, 41, 43
grief, being admitted into care example, 102
group working, 108–9
guidelines
    Action on Hearing Loss, 57–8
    dealing with difficult people, 107–8
    *see also* codes of practice
guilt, 81

Harris, T., 74
hearing-impaired people, 57–8, 103
hello greetings, 41
homelessness, 79
homophobia, 25, 55
hope, 27
hopelessness, 91–2
hunger, 21, 103, 104
Hunter, J., 5
hygiene, personal, 46–7, 51

identity formation, 26
illness/disability, living with, 78, 81, 87
I'm OK, You're OK life position, 73–5, *74*
important things, 99–101
information source, transmission model,
        *11*, 12
inner processes, 35
    Borton's development framework, 31–2
    further reading, 35–6
    intrapersonal communication, viii,
        19–20
    negative thinking, 27–9
    positive thinking, 28, 29
    reflective practice, 29–35
    self-awareness, 20–7
    SWOT analysis, *30*
    three-step reflective cycle, 32–5, *33*
Institute of Management Excellence, 104–5
integrity, 24
intercultural communication, 51–7
internal impacts on the self
    barriers to effective communication, 103
    self-awareness, 23–7
International Transactional Analysis Association
        (TAA), 61–2
interpersonal communication, viii, 37, 58
    cultural perspectives, 51–7, 58
    deaf/hearing-impaired people, 57–8
    environmental communication, 49–51, 58
    further reading, 59–60
    interpersonal skills, 38–9
    non-verbal communication, *45*, 45–9,
        *47*, 58
    paralanguage, 44–5
    verbal communication, 39–44, 58
    *see also* listening to people
interpreters, language barriers, 56–7
intrapersonal communication, viii, 19–20
invisible and unvoiced differences, cultural
        perspectives, 54

invisible and voiced differences, cultural
    perspectives, 54
isolation, listening to people, 78

joined-up thinking, 109
journal-keeping, 22

Kabat-Zinn, J., 22
knowing one's limitations, 22–3; *see also*
    self-awareness

language
    ego states, 64, 65, 66, 68
    intercultural communication, 51, 52, 53,
        55–7
    interpersonal communication, 38, 39–40,
        40, 43
    meanings, 14
    subjective understanding of, 14, 38, 40, 58
life positions/scripts, Transactional Analysis,
    73–5, *74*
limitations, knowing, 22–3; *see also* self-
    awareness
LinkedIn, 113
listening to people, viii–ix, 95–6
    active listening, 85–94, 96
    communication through listening, 77–80
    confidentiality, 94–5, 96
    dealing with difficult people, 105
    empathy, 80–1, 85, 87, 88, 95
    further reading, 96–7
    genuineness, 83–4, 95, 96
    self-disclosure, 84–5
    unconditional positive regard, 82–3
Littlejohn, S. W., 6
living with illness/disability, 78, 81, 87
loneliness, 78
looking closer, three-step reflective cycle, 32,
    *33*, 34
loss, being admitted into care example, 102

master aptitude, 27
meanings, creating, 6, 13–15
mechanistic frameworks, theories of
    communication, 10, *11*, 11–13
Mehrabian, A., 45, *45*
mental illness, 78
mentors, 22
Mid Staffordshire NHS Foundation
    Trust, 2
mind over matter, 66

mindfulness-based cognitive therapy (MBC),
    21–2, 27
models of communication, 10–16, *11*, *14*
modes of communication, 4, 8–9
    email, ix, 9, 110, 112–13
    telephone communication, 8, 9, 10, 110,
        111–12
    text messages, ix, 4, 9, 110, 112–13
    written communication, 110–11, 114
Moss, B., 95
musts, parent ego state, 64

names, 41–2
natural child ego state, 68
negative thinking, 27–9
Nelson Jones, R., 82
networking, 109
*NHS Knowledge and Skills Framework* (NHS
    Employers), 3, 5
NHS Records Management Code of Practice,
    109
NHS Social Media Toolkit, 113
noise
    barriers to effective communication, 103
    models of communication, *11*, 12–13, 15
non-judgemental positive regard, 38, 82–3, 96
non-malevolence (not harming), 24
non-verbal communication, 39, *45*, 45–9, *47*,
    51, 58
    active listening, 91
    environmental communication, 49–51
    *see also* body language
non-verbal de-escalation, dealing with difficult
    people, 108
Nursing and Midwifery Council Code of
    Conduct (2012), 94

Oelofsen, N., 32–5, *33*
Office for National Statistics Census 2011,
    55–6
OK life position, 73–5, *74*
open questions, 90–1, 94, 107
opportunities, SWOT analysis, *30*
optimism, 27
others, definition, 4

paralanguage, 44–5, 65
paraphrasing, active listening, 88–9, 90, 93
parent ego state, 62, 63–5, 68–9, *70*, *71*,
    *72*, 75
    dealing with difficult people, 106, *107*

patient satisfaction, non-verbal communication, 46
peer groups, 26
personal hygiene, 46–7, 51
personal values, *see* values
personality dragons, 104–5
person-centred therapy, 79–80
pet names, 42
physical needs
    external impacts on the self, 20–1
    listening to people, 81
Piaget, J., 65
positive regard, 38, 82–3, 96
positive thinking, 28, 29
posture, 47, *47*, 51, 58, 86
practical application, ix, 114
    barriers to effective communication, 103–4, 114
    codes of practice, 109–10, 114
    dealing with difficult people, 104–8, *107*
    email/text, 112–13
    further reading, 114–15
    most important things to people, 99–101
    self-awareness, 101–2, 106, 114
    social media, 113
    telephone communication, 110, 111–12
    working in partnership, 108–9, 114
    written communication, 110–11, 114
preferred way of being, 74
prospective reflection, 29
psychological frameworks for theories of communication, 11; *see also* transactional model

questioning, 90–1, 94

race, cultural perspectives, 53
rationality, adult ego state, 65–6
reading activities, ix
    being admitted into care case study, 119
    communication, 3
    dealing with difficult people, 104
    Transactional Analysis, 75
receivers, models of communication, *11*, 12, *14*
record-keeping, written communication, 110–11
red card, symbolism of, 6–7
reflections, x
    appropriate methods of communication, 9
    dealing with difficult people, 105–6
    external impacts on the self, 22
    intercultural communication, 54, 55, 56

interpersonal communication, 37, 41, 43, 45, 46, 51
    listening to people, 78, 81, 82, 83
    most important things to people, 99–100
    negative thinking, 28
    noise, 12
    self-awareness, 101–2
    symbols, 6, 7
    Transactional Analysis, 66, 73
    values, 25, 26
reflective practice, 29–35, 87–8, 93
reframing, negative thinking, 28
residential care home example
    barriers to effective communication, 104
    Borton's development framework, 31–2
    three-step reflective cycle, 33–4
respectfulness, 24, 95, 118
retrospective reflection, 29
Rogers, C., 23, 38, 77, 79–80, 83, 122

scripts, Transactional Analysis, 73–5, *74*
self-awareness, 20–7, 114
    body language, 86–7
    dealing with difficult people, 106, 114
    external impacts on the self, 20–3
    internal impacts on the self, 23–7
    practical application, 101–2
    reflective practice, 30, 32
self-concepts, 101
self-disclosure, 84–5
self-esteem, 55, 82, 101, 114
self-talk, 19, 27, 29
Serious Case Review of Daniel Pelka, 57
sexuality, cultural perspectives, 53
Shannon and Weaver transmission model, *11*, 11–13, 15, 103
shoulds/shouldn'ts, parent ego state, 64
silence, active listening, 91, 94
sincerity, 24
6 Cs, core values and behaviours, 2
smoking example, ego states, 66–7
social constructionist frameworks for theories of communication, 11; *see also* transactional model
social grraacceess acronym, 53
social media, ix, 9, 112, 113
socioeconomic class, 53
spirituality, cultural perspectives, 53
Mr Spock, *Star Trek*, 65
stereotyped views, 53, 58

strengths, SWOT analysis, *30*
structural analysis, ego states, 62
subjective understanding of language, 14, 38, 40, 58
suicidal thoughts, active listening, 91–2, 94
summarising, active listening, 89–90, 93
SWOT (strengths, weaknesses, opportunities, threats) analysis, *30*
symbols, 6–7, 14, 52
systemic frameworks for theories of communication, 11; *see also* transactional model
systemic family therapy, 53

TA, *see* Transactional Analysis
telephone communication, 8, 9, 10, 110, 111–12
text messages, ix, 4, 9, 110, 112–13
therapeutic relationship, 47, 53, 85
threats, SWOT analysis, *30*
three-step (CLT) reflective cycle, 32–5, *33*, 104
tiredness, 20, 21, 81
    barriers to effective communication, 103, 104
    external impacts on the self, 21
tone of voice/tonality
    ego states, 64, 65, 66, 68
    non-verbal communication, 45, *45* , 52
    *see also* paralanguage
touch, 49, 51
traffic symbols, 7
Transactional Analysis Association (TAA), 61–2
Transactional Analysis (TA), viii, 27, 61–2, 76
    complementary transactions, 69–70, *70*
    crossed transactions, *71*, 71–2
    ego states, 62–9
    further reading, 76
    life scripts, 73–5, *74*
    ulterior or covert transactions, 72, *72*
transactional model of communication, 11, 13–16, *14*
transformation, three-step reflective cycle, 33, *33*, 34
transitions, *see* change/transition
transmission model, Shannon and Weaver, *11*, 11–13, 15, 103
transmitters, models of communication, *11*, 12, *14*
trustworthiness, 24

truthfulness, 24
Twitter, 113

ulterior transactions, 72, *72*
unconditional positive regard, 38, 82–3, 96
understanding ourselves, *see* self-awareness

values, 5
    barriers to effective communication, 103
    core, 6 Cs, 2
    internal impacts on the self, 23–7
verbal communication, 39–44, 58
verbal de-escalation, dealing with difficult people, 107–8
visible and unvoiced differences, cultural perspectives, 54
visible and voiced differences, cultural perspectives, 53–4
voice tone, *see* tone of voice/tonality
Vygotsky, L. S., 24

warmth, 38, 82–3
weaknesses, SWOT analysis, *30*
Weaver, W., *see* Shannon and Weaver transmission model
wellbeing, 104, 114
    and communication, 5
    and listening to people, 78, 85, 96
*What is Transactional Analysis? A personal and practical guide* (Whitton), 73
Wood, J., 5, 6, 7
    transactional model of communication, 13–16, *14*
words used, ego states, 64, 65, 66, 68; *see also* language
working in partnership, 108–9, 114
writing activities, x
    active listening, 92–3, 94
    barriers to effective communication, 103
    definitions of communication, 3–8
    interpersonal skills, 38–9
    modes of communication, 8, 9
    SWOT analysis, 31
    three-step reflective cycle, 35
    Transactional Analysis, 64, 68, 73
written communication, 110–11, 114